Dr. Jettli
Dr Sancar

GOODBYE,
PILLS & NEEDLES:

A Total Re-Think of Type II Diabetes
And A 90 Day Cure

By Tom Jelinek, PhD

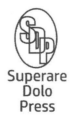

Superare
Dolo
Press

Important Disclaimer

CONTENTS

About The Author

Tom Jelinek earned his PhD in 1993 (McMaster University), studying cellular regulatory processes. He then joined the Cancer Center at the University of Virginia Medical School, where he furthered his studies on the mechanisms of cell signaling. Growth factors or other hormones hit their receptors on cells, which initiate biochemical signals inside those cells, and control physiological processes. One growth factor receptor of interest was the insulin-like growth factor receptor. It is peripherally involved in many cancers, is highly similar to the insulin receptor, and a high dose of insulin will activate both receptors. After leaving the University of Virginia, Tom spent 15 years in a strategic role in biotechnology, where it was essential to keep abreast of all significant developments.

At age 51, Tom was diagnosed with type II diabetes, with a blood glucose reading of 325 mg/dl (18 mM). But instead of turning to medication, he returned to his roots, and began to ask what went wrong, and whether it could be cured by reversing what went wrong. The result was a halving of blood glucose in under a month, and full reversal of diabetes in under three months. He spent the next three years questioning, dissecting, and re-thinking every aspect of diabetes. Along the way, it became clear that diabetes treatment orthodoxy is a derivative of the same orthodoxy that gave us the *food pyramid*, replacing fat with carbohydrates, ostensibly to prevent heart disease. The advice has produced the exact opposite of what was promised, and yet the guidelines remain in place. Seeing the public health disaster unfolding in front of him, Tom decided it is time for the world to hear why those guidelines caused the diabetes epidemic, and how it can easily be fixed.

Preface

The doctor of the future will give no medicine but will interest his patients in the care of the human frame, in diet and in the cause and prevention of disease. ~ Thomas Edison

It is one thing to master a discipline. It is another thing entirely to live it, and subject one's life to its maxims. For me, it began in earnest when I saw the reading of 18 mM blood glucose (325 mg/dl). I was advised on the spot to see an endocrinologist, who would find the right combination of drugs to treat my diabetes. I briefly felt sick to the stomach, as I confronted the facts. I then began to question the whole premise. *Combinations of drugs? Aren't there better options?* I had given mainstream dietary guidelines the benefit of the doubt until that moment, and it ended badly. What if diabetes treatment guidelines were equally wrong?

My brain is wired to think of life through the *eyes* of individual cells, and to see the organism as the sum of its cells. I knew my blood glucose was too high, and it was slowly poisoning me. My muscle cells were refusing to take it out of circulation. Probably my liver, also. Should I override those refusals with diabetes drugs? That didn't feel right, so I tried the only other option: To stop eating anything that could raise my blood glucose. In short, carbohydrates. I never again ate potatoes, bread, or any other starchy food. I have not had a drop of beer, or any sweet drink. Not even fruit juice. I acted first, and asked questions later. Right or wrong, I had to follow my instincts. A decision on drugs could come later, if all else failed.

Fortunately, all else did not fail. Within three weeks, my blood glucose had come down from 325 mg/dl to under 150 mg/dl. Within three months, my morning blood glucose was below 100 mg/dl as often as it was slightly above. In the afternoon, I average about 90 mg/dl. If measured for the first time today, depending on the day, I would be considered normal, or *post-diabetic*. I coined that term, to describe myself. *Pre-diabetic* implies an inevitability I have since come to reject. My other symptoms have all faded, and my health is as good as ever. I am no longer drowsy in the afternoon. I can hike for many hours without lagging, and I am deeply grateful for my new lease on life.

It quickly became clear that the medical system looks at diabetes purely in terms of controlling blood glucose, making it the only objective, regardless what it does to the cells tasked with taking it out of the blood. Medicine is very eager to treat the many complications of diabetes, but is not so eager to suggest the one course of action that can stop it in its tracks: Avoidance of carbs. And in spite of all the interventions, the official outlook is bleak. Many doctors and researchers refer to diabetics as *the walking dead*. Once blood glucose regulation goes off, they say, the *horses have left the barn*. Our life expectancy is TEN YEARS less than others', due principally to what is called our *extraordinarily high risk of heart disease*. And what about drugs? Six large trials on type II diabetics tried to establish that blood glucose reduction with drugs could improve cardiovascular disease risk. Every one failed, so they upped the doses, and tried again. The result? A significantly *increased* risk of death in the treatment group (Byington et. al., NEJM 2008; 358:2545-2559). To call those treatment strategies ineffective would be to flatter them. They can make things a lot worse. Yet somehow, most doctors missed the reports that drugs can make things worse, and continue to prescribe those same drugs. Understandably, the drug reps did not enthusiastically spread that news.

For me, low-carb living is all it took to break insulin resistance, the molecular cause of type II diabetes. There are plenty of good resources available to support low-carb dieting, but they are targeted principally to weight loss. Without a support system, I experienced several crises of confidence, which might have put me off my approach, were I not so stubborn. I learned how difficult it is to openly defy the guidelines pushed by the medical system. It was always a burden to see the incredulous expression, every time I told a medical professional I was reducing my blood glucose by avoiding dietary sources of glucose. It felt like they were thinking, "You just relax. We'll call the nice people with the padded wagon, and have them take you home." A brief lecture, and a handout explaining the dietary guidelines was always the response. Seeing no alternative, I made it my mission to understand diabetes in-depth, and as a result, developed confidence that I was on the right path.

Along the way, I was inspired by the example of William Banting, who first popularized low-carb dieting. After years of fruitless struggle with his weight, he lost enormous amounts of weight when he cut out the carbs, and felt an obligation to share his success as widely as he could. In 1863, he published his *Letter on Corpulence*, for that purpose. Now, like Banting, I feel an obligation to share my experiences and my understanding of what goes wrong in diabetes, and how it is cured.

The standard advice embodied in the food pyramid brought us to where a third of all Americans are either diabetic, or well on their way to being diabetic. That's 100 million people, in America alone. If each of us were to lose ten years of life, that's a loss of one billion people-years. Clearly, the standard approach is not working. And when something does the exact opposite of what we want, it's a logical imperative to invert it, if only to see if that achieves improved results. For me, it obviously did, and now I'd like to tell the world why it worked so well.

Structure: Part one consists of a re-thinking of type II diabetes, from the ground up. The disease has little in common with type I diabetes, apart from hyperglycemia, yet the medical system treats it as though it were the same disease. This error is deconstructed, and a new model is put forth, of type II diabetes as a nutritional problem, caused by a chronic overuse of insulin, leading to the runaway insulin resistance feedback loop. The perfect diet to break that feedback loop is a high fat, low carb diet, the science of which is also reviewed. Finally, the single biggest reason why every diabetic is not already using a high fat low carb diet is because of their fears of heart disease. Others have conclusively disproven this myth, and I review those works, and examine the true causes (plural) of heart disease.

In part two, I review what it is like to live the theory, what misconceptions and mistakes I had to overcome, and what a person should expect when curing oneself of type II diabetes. Unfortunately, a supportive medical system is not something to expect, and I call on physicians and other medical professionals to take note that this works, and assist patients as they make this same journey. I also cover additional things I learned about diabetes after the fact, including the role of chronic stress in its causation. I conclude with a call to hold advice accountable, whether it comes from a book, or from a government committee. When it fails, acknowledge that it failed, and discard it. Diabetics' lives are on the line, and time is of the essence. Waiting for guidelines to change is not an option.

Part three consists of resources I compiled over the past three years. Rather than present a cookbook, I share my tips to transform your favorite dishes into low-carb alternatives. Only by approximating what you've always eaten can you sustain a diet in the long run. I include a review of existing diabetes drugs and supplements, and their mechanisms of action. I moved them out of the main text once I concluded it was best not to use them.

Scientific Terminology: I've made a concerted effort to make this book readable for those with only introductory scientific literacy. I tested it on a college freshman biology student, who claimed it was fine. Nonetheless, there may be sections too scientific for some: Chapter 2 in particular, where carbohydrate metabolism is reviewed. I felt it important to include this chapter nonetheless, to lay the groundwork for the rest of the book. For those who find it too much, simply skim over it, and feel free to return to it when questions arise.

Documentation: There is a reasonable expectation that extraordinary claims should be backed up by something other than the writer's say-so. And yet it is common to find references cited selectively to support a particular approach, while contradictory references are ignored. Furthermore, the evidence presented in those papers often fails to match the claims made by the one citing them. This problem is compounded by cases where the title of a paper appears to contradict the data presented. The most likely culprit is a journal editor, shy about contradicting an established consensus. The outcome is that one can no longer trust a work simply because it includes many references.

I deal with this issue in a manner similar to Malcolm Kendrick, to whose work I refer in several places. When addressing a specific trial, I cite that trial. When addressing a claim, I refer to the source that makes the claim. When it comes to scientific minutiae, I cite relevant review articles, but I do not review each piece of primary research. When questions arise, I invite the reader to conduct their own search (https://www.ncbi.nlm.nih.gov/pubmed/), to see the full complexity of work that could be interpreted as relevant.

PART ONE: Overturning Conventional Wisdom

Introduction

Sickness is the discord of the elements infused into the body ~ Leonardo da Vinci

Medical practice imagines insulin like a rheostat, whose principal function is to reduce glucose in the blood following a carb-rich meal. When that rheostat goes wrong, the practitioner tinkers with it, to try to *fix* it. There's an implicit understanding that insulin resistance is a malfunction to be fixed, rather than a natural response to be respected. Most diabetes drugs are designed to do precisely that.

But what if that understanding of insulin is all wrong? What if chronically elevated insulin is the problem, rather than the solution? Let me pose a question, by way of introducing the topic. What do you consider the single biggest threat to your life? Many who've read this far might answer, "The complications of diabetes; foremost among them, heart disease." From our modern perspective, I'd have to agree. But today's diseases were exceedingly rare only a hundred years ago. Sure, we live longer today, due to antibiotics and clean water, but increases in our age fail to explain the severity of the diabetes epidemic, which is now reducing overall life expectancy.

Increased consumption of refined sugar and carbohydrates match the rise of diabetes, so they're obviously suspects. But carbohydrates have been a staple food for thousands of years. Why are they suddenly be causing us so much harm? After all, the refinement of sugars and carbohydrates does not create any new metabolic processes. It merely increases the glucose load after a meal (and increases fructose). Could we be so sensitive to carbohydrates that a mere increase in their potency would make us so sick?

If we were meant to live principally on carbohydrates, we would surely be resistant to harm even from their refined versions. But if our biochemistry was optimized for a different diet, and the makeup of our diet changed radically in recent history, the implications change. If raw carbohydrates were only a seasonal food for our ancestors, then the switch to an endless diet of refined carbohydrates could be enough to push us over the edge. And if we remember that farming is a recent historical development, the link between carbs and diabetes needs to be considered.

The sudden rise of farming is often called the *Neolithic Revolution*. As the name implies, it was a radical change from hunting and gathering every food that was available. But our genes, and the programs they encode, do not change the moment people make a fundamental lifestyle change. By and large, our genes are the same as when our ancestors were hunter-gatherers.

Now, let's re-direct the question I initially posed: What were the biggest threats to the lives of our hunter-gatherer ancestors? Getting eaten by lions, or gored by buffalo, would certainly be threats. As would infections, plagues, and tribal warfare. But those are not predictable, and nutrition can't change them. It was in fact starvation that posed the single biggest predictable threat they faced. And especially in temperate climates, they faced extreme seasonal variations in the diversity and quantity of available food. Even people in warm climates faced seasonal variations in their food supply.

Fortunately for our ancestors, the winter was preceded by a time of plenty. Fruits ripened on trees, root vegetables were at their richest, and to the extent that grains were a part of the diet, those also ripened at that time. So it was essential to their survival to store away as many calories as possible, during that short time of plenty. This is a departure from the simple equilibrium between energy intake and expenditure that is ordinarily in place. Autumn was a special time, a primordial *Oktoberfest*, where equilibrium was tossed aside, so maximum fat reserves could be built up. Many animals do this. The difference is they continue to live that way today, whereas our lifestyle has undergone a radical change.

To make use of the excess calories available in the fall, it's essential that our genes encode a program to maximize calorie storage during that time of plenty. If we had to invent that program today, we would mandate that it respond to the presence of excess glucose (the seasonal fuel), and divert most of it to the liver, where it can be converted to fat, then shuttled off and stored in adipocytes. It would have to make the person chronically hungry and lethargic, to ensure maximal food consumption and minimal physical activity,

10

ensuring all excess calories are used to build stockpiles of fat. It would have to shut down the leptin signal, whereby fat cells tell the brain, "We're full, so stop eating. Go off and chase buffalo, or whatever it is cavemen do for amusement."

This exact program exists. We refer to it as *insulin*. We simply think of insulin as a blood glucose regulator because hyperglycemia (high blood glucose) is the most striking manifestation of its loss, in type I diabetes. But insulin reduces blood glucose incidentally, as part of its primary function: To build fat reserves.

Nearly all life functions are tightly regulated, to ensure all the parts act in coordinated fashion to support the needs of the whole. And most regulation happens through negative feedback loops, where any disruption of equilibrium is met with responses designed to quickly restore that equilibrium. For instance, you're low on energy, you get hungry, you eat, you now have sufficient energy, you're not hungry anymore. Very few processes are regulated by positive feedback, where each round of the cycle amplifies the previous one. And those that are tend to end in some highly decisive fashion. For instance, the contractions involved in childbirth are self-reinforcing, until the baby is born. But insulin resistance is also an example of positive feedback. It is a natural response, and it is programmed into our genes, to help us avoid starvation.

In brief, the spike in blood glucose that follows the consumption of fruits, starchy vegetables, and grains triggers insulin secretion, which initially signals the muscles and liver to take up glucose, and store some of it in the form of glycogen. Those stores are eventually filled, and if glucose continues to be in excess, it is in the interests of the body to divert it to the liver, for conversion to fat. So how do you get more glucose to go to the liver? The easiest way is for the muscles to become insulin resistant. They're happy to oblige, once they've filled their glycogen stores.

Insulin resistance only builds from there. Fructose, the sweet sub-unit of sucrose and HFCS, is only taken up by the liver, and in amounts above about 50 grams at once, overloads the liver's capacity to burn it as fuel. It cannot be stored, so it is converted to fat. Once new fat builds to a certain level, some of it makes it to the muscles. If it arrives while glucose remains in excess, it is a sure signal that food is abundant. It's time to make fat, and the muscles respond by ramping up insulin resistance.

Increasing insulin resistance in muscles, while the carb feast continues, results in elevated blood glucose levels, and leads to ever more insulin production. That insulin signal increasingly focuses on the liver and fat cells, with the muscles now insulin resistant. In the liver, all the extra glucose is converted to fat. The newly synthesized fat causes ever more insulin resistance, more insulin secretion, and more fat synthesis. Fat eventually builds up in the liver, causing inflammation and insulin resistance in that organ. The feedback loop has the potential to spiral out of control, but for one thing: The season of plenty ends after a short time, and the fuel runs out. Winter sets in, glucose becomes scarce, and all the signals are turned off quickly enough. Over the course of the winter, equilibrium is restored, and fat is burned off.

But what happens when the season of plenty is extended indefinitely? There is no dispute that excess glucose is toxic in the blood, due to its reactivity with the body's proteins (the basis for the HbA1C test). But the potential for damage is even greater inside cells, where oxidative damage caused by the reaction of glucose with proteins in the cell, can kill that cell. So eventually, the cells of the liver cannot process glucose quickly enough, and are threatened by the excess glucose they are tasked with taking up. They respond by also becoming insulin resistant. That's not a malfunction. Cells are programmed to react in this way, and are triggered by a side-pathway for glucose metabolism. It senses glucose concentration, and when too high, it inhibits the insulin response. With the liver now also insulin resistant, blood glucose rises sharply, and ever increasing levels of insulin secretion and insulin resistance follow, until the pancreatic beta cells hit their limit. Insulin, already extremely high, can go no higher, to force reluctant cells to take up the constant excess of glucose. That's when we call it type II diabetes.

Today, medicine steps in, and overrides cells' refusal to take up excess glucose, with varying degrees of success, as judged against the narrowly defined measure of blood glucose levels. But the outcome is toxicity for liver cells, escalating insulin resistance, hyper secretion of insulin leading to pancreatic burnout, worsening high blood pressure, and elevated heart disease risk.

So what if instead of trying to stuff ever more glucose into cells, we did what our ancestors did, before insulin resistance could cause serious damage. What if we cut off the fuel of the positive feedback loop? All it takes is to voluntarily stop consuming carbohydrates. Could we achieve the same restoration of equilibrium as our ancestors did, during their long winters? Can we break the positive feedback loop, and reset the system? Based on my personal experience doing exactly that, my answer is *yes, absolutely.*

Chapter 1: Re-Thinking Diabetes

Time and time again, throughout the history of medical practice, what was once considered scientific *eventually becomes regarded as* bad practice. ~ David Stewart

The Establishment View

If you believe the official story, including the stance of the American Diabetes Association, diabetes is caused by dietary fat. This is based on the observation that muscle cells grown in a dish and fed fat are insulin resistant. But dietary fat spends very little time in the blood, especially in diabetics, whose astronomical insulin levels ensure it is quickly stored in adipocytes, and never released. It is only when dietary carbs are in chronic excess, causing the liver to spew out huge quantities of fat, that both fat and carbs are in circulation for an extended time. So it's new fat, made by the liver from carbs, that triggers muscle cell insulin resistance. And it's highly reversible, if the carbs are cut off. But blaming dietary fat conforms to the dictates of the anti-fat crusade of the 1970s and 1980s. To put the question to rest, let's review a couple of key facts, and decide for ourselves.

First, consider the Inuit people of the Arctic. Their traditional diets rely very much on seal and whale blubber for calories, supplemented with whatever other parts of the animal they eat. They don't know diabetes, and their heart disease rates are very low. Unless, that is, they convert to a diet of imported, processed food rich in carbs. Then, they quickly come down with obesity and severe diabetes. Further, it can easily be reversed, by going back to the traditional diet, high in fat [Described in the documentary *My Big Fat Diet*, by Sally Norris]. Is that compatible with the idea that fat causes diabetes?

The Inuit are only one people, living in an extreme environment with no history of agriculture, so let's consider what happened across North America over the past forty years. The anti-fat crusade was formally launched by the McGovern Commission in the late 1970s, and we were exhorted to reduce our fat consumption from 40% of total calories, to 30%. We were promised a reduction in heart disease rates if we complied. And we complied. The people of the United States did exactly as they were told, and reduced fat consumption to 30% of calories. This neutralizes any arguments claiming a lack of compliance with guidelines. You have to eat something, however, so carbs took the place of fat, as those on the commission knew would happen. As for the stated objective of the recommendations, the reduction of heart disease? Heart disease rates went through the roof. Obesity rates skyrocketed, especially for children. And the incidence of diabetes exploded. Tripled, and the trend suggests it is far from over. Fat consumption fell and diabetes rates tripled, but the ADA continues to say that fat causes diabetes. In doing so, they forfeit the right to claim leadership on the issue.

The Hippocratic Oath is often summarized as an obligation of the physician to, *First, do no harm.* It is no longer routine for physicians to take the oath, but the principle remains one to which we should hold the medical establishment. In judging the process that gave us our dietary guidelines, the only possible verdict is that it failed the Hippocratic principle. It would be wrong to keep trusting that process, without extensive scrutiny.

While it would be nice if the guidelines were changed to stop actively harming public health, this may always be an uphill battle. Guidelines affect many things besides individual health, including the profitability of food and drug makers, the subsidies given to certain foods for the poor, or for school lunches, agricultural subsidies, and even environmental concerns regarding agricultural practices. Any political process that aims to change guidelines has to hear from all those interests. And even if an overwhelming case were made, and heard, there would be so many objections that more time is needed to make adjustments, that those of us already diabetic will be long dead before anything changes. But change can happen at the individual level. The numbers of doctors who have discovered the truth are growing, and each of them can influence many patients. Informed patients are demanding that the medical system respond to their needs, rather than simply write ineffective prescriptions. It is my hope to accelerate that process, so that one day, the political process will have no choice but to acknowledge the reality that type II diabetes is a dietary disease, with a dietary cure.

Summary: Official organs say fat causes diabetes, but that's provably wrong. Inuit eating fat do not know diabetes unless they switch to carbohydrates. When recommendations were made to switch to carbs, we cut our fat, increased carbs, and diabetes rates went through the roof. Official organs failed the Hippocratic principle to do no harm.

The Breakthrough, The Error

Diabetes was first described in ancient Egypt, although it was considered rare. It tended to strike the young very suddenly, and their condition could deteriorate quickly, ending in death. One early observation was that the urine of diabetics would attract ants, because of the glucose it contained. In fifth century India, it was first observed that overweight adults could develop a similar disease, characterized by glucose in the urine, leading to its recognition as a separate disorder. But the cause remained elusive.

In 1922, Frederick Banting and Charles Best first purified insulin, and showed it was the factor missing from those with juvenile diabetes (today called type I diabetes). Those lacking insulin died, whereas those who received injections of insulin thrived. That ranks insulin among the most transformative of all medical discoveries. And because it was such a breakthrough, it defined how we think of diabetes. We concluded that insulin was the natural factor that cleared glucose from the blood. From there, it was very easy to make a lazy leap in medical thinking, and decide that the *only* function of insulin is to clear glucose from the blood. When that error informs the objectives of treating diabetes, we end up attempting to stuff glucose into cells in any way possible.

The following table compares type I and type II diabetes. Do you see many similarities?

Diabetes	Insulin	Blood Glucose	Body Fat	BHB (ketone)
Type I	None	Very high, quickly	Very low	Dangerously high
Type II	Very High	Climbs slowly	High	None

The traditional understanding of insulin as a glucose uptake regulator remains relevant for type I diabetes, even if it is incomplete. Type I diabetics tend to be emaciated (very little body fat), and produce excessive amounts of the blood ketone beta hydroxybutyrate (BHB). Those are the symptoms of starvation, even while blood glucose is highly elevated. Insulin regulates all three. Type II diabetes, however, is far more common among the overweight, and the ketone BHB is not normally produced. Furthermore, type II diabetics produce excessive amounts of insulin. In fact, the only thing common to the two diseases is high blood glucose, and even there, the course of the disease is very much different. And yet, the terminology of type I versus type II diabetes speaks to how we consider them subsets of the same disease, in need of the same treatment strategies.

The very strong association of type II diabetes with weight gain, high blood pressure, and high triglycerides relative to HDL strongly suggests one common cause. They were once called Syndrome X, and today Metabolic Syndrome. And the defining feature is that in spite of high to very high blood insulin levels, blood glucose is also high because of insulin resistance. The conventional medical thinking holds that the objective of treatment is to overcome insulin resistance, or find a way around it, in order to force cells to take up excess glucose, and clear it from the blood. In other words, it remains only an extension of the thinking on type I diabetes, where the insulin signal is missing entirely.

While diabetes is narrowly defined as hyperglycemia, the complications that come with type II diabetes are caused by a combination of chronically high blood glucose, and the elevated insulin levels that accompany it. In other words, rising insulin levels are part of the problem, and raising them even further will worsen the problem. Chronically elevated insulin causes fluid retention, and vascular smooth muscle cell hypertrophy. Those are the muscles that wrap around arteries, and when overdeveloped, they squeeze harder, and don't give as much with each pulse. Add to that increased fluid volume in the circulatory system, and blood pressure rises very high.

Elevated insulin also raises the risk of cancer. Cells that have no insulin receptors do not become insulin resistant, and yet they are also targets of elevated insulin. The insulin-like growth factor-I

(IGF-I) receptor is on all cell types, and it can be activated by elevated concentrations of insulin. We used insulin instead of IGF-I when studying the IGF-I receptor in the laboratory, because insulin was far cheaper, and could do the job perfectly well, if we used an elevated dose. In the body, insulin also boosts free IGF-I levels, by knocking it off specialized proteins that keep it tied up and inactive. And there is a sizeable body of research outlining the contributory role played by the IGF-I receptor in the development of many types of cancer.

Given these dangers of excessive insulin, what if we began to think of insulin in a new way? Instead of thinking of insulin as the hormone that clears glucose from the blood, recognize it for what we now know it is: The principal signal for the body to put on weight, using a short-lived excess of available glucose to build up fat reserves. If we do this, we will see insulin resistant diabetes not as a technical obstacle to overcome, but as an innate physiologic response to too much glucose consumption, on a chronic basis. And our treatment strategy will be radically different than it is today.

Summary: When insulin is lacking entirely, in type I diabetes, the patient shows the signs of starvation, even with high blood glucose. When insulin is in excess, in type II diabetes, the patient is usually overweight. The two are different diseases, and need to be treated differently. If type I diabetes is caused by too little insulin, type II diabetes could be considered a disease of too much insulin. The solution is not even more insulin, but less need of insulin.

Other Hormones That Regulate Blood Glucose

Insulin is far from the only hormone that has an affect on blood glucose levels. Glucagon is produced by the alpha cells of the pancreas, by contrast with insulin, which is produced by the beta cells. Glucagon stimulates the breakdown of glycogen in the liver, causing glucose release. Once the liver's glycogen is depleted, glucagon also stimulates production of new glucose from broken down proteins. In healthy individuals, the alpha cells are suppressed by insulin, and glucagon production is kept under control, unless glucose levels fall, and insulin goes quiet. But in type II diabetes, insulin resistance extends to the alpha cells, resulting in elevated glucagon production, and elevated glucose production by the liver, even in the face of excess glucose in the blood. In type I diabetes, where no insulin is present, no signal is delivered to the alpha cells, to stop glucagon production. The result is also overproduction of glucose by the liver. Accordingly, some amount of hyperglycemia, both in type I and type II diabetes, is due to excessive glucagon production, leading to excessive glucose production by the liver.

A second hormone that boosts blood glucose is cortisol, the stress hormone. It is a steroid hormone that changes gene expression patterns in the liver, resulting in more glucose production. Cortisol has many other properties besides boosting glucose, and chronically elevated cortisol is implicated in disorders from diabetes to heart disease. Later, faulty regulation of cortisol is discussed as a contributory factor to both diseases.

Incretins (GLP-1, GIP) are hormones that stimulate the secretion of insulin after a meal, before the blood glucose spike fully sets in, as well as inhibiting the production of glucagon. Additionally, they slow the rate of stomach emptying, and probably decrease food intake as a result. Once in circulation, incretins are rapidly degraded by dipeptidyl peptidase-4 (DPP-4). As a result, they only spend a minute or two in circulation, before equilibrium begins to be restored. A new generation of diabetes drugs increases incretin levels by inhibiting DPP-4, thus causing more insulin to be released, for longer intervals.

Amylin (or Islet Amyloid Polypeptide - IAPP), like insulin, is produced by the beta cells of the pancreas, at a rate directly proportional to insulin (about 1:100 of amylin: insulin). The two genes share what is called a promoter element, meaning that increased production of one always comes together with the other. Amylin slows the emptying of the stomach, and increases satiety. It also plays a role in the inhibition of glucagon production. As such, it plays a minor role in the regulation of blood glucose. But in type II diabetes, as insulin levels rise in an attempt to overcome insulin resistance, amylin levels rise at precisely the same rate. At a certain point, more amylin is made than can be properly processed by the beta cells (the functional form has parts precisely chopped off by specialized enzymes, and at high levels, they can't keep up), and the unprocessed form of amylin accumulates. Given enough accumulation, it can form globs, called amyloid, that are thought to cause the death of beta cells characteristic of the late stages of type II diabetes. At that point, the patient must take insulin injections.

Finally, it is likely that all the players have not yet been described, and of those that are known, some will prove to have additional functions. One intriguing observation is that in some cases, patients with type II diabetes who have had parts of their duodenum removed for various medical reasons, were no longer diabetic after the surgery. In other cases, bypass of the duodenum and jejunum reversed type II diabetes. The mechanism is not understood, but the *anti-incretin theory* suggests that a factor produced in the upper small intestine can interfere with glucose control. An inflammatory cytokine could easily fit the description.

Should we try to cure diabetes with surgery? I don't think so. Tonsils and adenoids were once routinely removed, until their role in the immune system was understood. So let's use this observation as a clue to look for a factor that regulates blood glucose, and not as justification for cutting out body parts.

Summary: Insulin is only one of many factors that affect blood glucose levels.

Leptin

There was considerable fanfare in the late 1990s, surrounding the discovery of leptin. It was reported as the factor missing from a strain of mice that were chronically lethargic, hungry, and obese. The reason for the excitement was obvious: Just as insulin was the missing factor in diabetes, leptin could be the missing factor in obesity. Rapidly increasing obesity in the general public over the past generation meant it was not a genetic change, but it was hoped injections of leptin could boost its signal, and cure obesity. It was the same rationale as is used to treat type II diabetes, by boosting the insulin signal.

When fat cells are satisfied, they make leptin. It is a hormone that travels through the blood to the brain, where it activates its receptor on the hypothalamus. The receptor initiates nerve signals that tell the body: I am not hungry, I have enough energy, and I can use it. A lack of leptin signals the opposite: I am hungry, I lack energy, and I don't want to waste any, exactly like that strain of mice that lacked a functioning leptin gene.

The excitement over leptin proved short-lived. The number of people lacking a functioning leptin gene is on the order of a dozen or two, in the whole world (and injections work very well for them). And leptin is made by adipocytes, rather than specialized cells like the beta cells of the pancreas. Obese people have high, even excessive, amounts of leptin. Like type II diabetics with high insulin levels, they are leptin resistant.

The mechanisms of leptin resistance turned out to be much simpler than those of insulin resistance. The culprit? Insulin. Every neuron that has leptin receptors also has insulin receptors. And whenever the two occur on the same cell, insulin blocks the leptin signal. So if a person is insulin sensitive, and only uses insulin in short pulses, after which it goes dormant again, leptin can do its job, and keep the person satisfied, and energetic. But when insulin is chronically elevated, leptin action is always blocked, and the person becomes hungry and lethargic all the time.

Everything comes back to that feast before winter, that our ancestors used in order to build fat reserves. When fat cells were adequately charged, they would ordinarily signal the brain to stop eating, and start chasing wild buffalo with spears. But if it was a carb feast at their disposal, then no chasing was necessary, or even desirable. It was time to put on as much fat as physically possible, and the food was right there to be had. So insulin did its work as the *get-fat* hormone, and blocked leptin, the *I've had enough* hormone from doing anything. The feast went on, and leptin could not stop it, until the carbs ran out.

Summary: Leptin is made by fat cells, telling the brain they're satisfied, and it's okay to be energetic, and stop eating. Excess insulin blocks leptin's signal, so the person is tired, hungry, and obese.

Inflammation and Insulin Resistance

Chronic inflammation is a cause of insulin resistance. Inflammation is typically initiated by hormones known as inflammatory cytokines. Their natural functions are often linked to getting an immune response started, and several are also made by fat cells. Among their many functions, inflammatory cytokines tell cells to shut off their insulin responses. To make a little sense out of this, consider that when fighting an infection, it does the body no good to be making fat from excess glucose. The pressing need is to fight the infection. The danger of starvation is farther off into the future. It might be better to let glucose levels rise a little, and give immune cells a little extra fuel. Or to feed a fever, which also plays an important role in fighting disease. My own experiences measuring my morning glucose numbers speak to this. Sometimes, I find my measurements up by 10% to 20%. Invariably, I get nervous, and wonder why this could be. I make a list of everything I ate, when I last exercised, and when those do not turn up an answer, I panic a little. Then, a day or two later, I develop the symptoms of a cold, and my glucose comes back down to its historic range. Then I breathe a sign of relief. It's a normal reaction to getting sick.

What about those inflammatory cytokines made by fat cells? The bigger the adipocyte, the higher the level of inflammatory cytokine production, again suggesting a positive feedback loop. I believe this to be a case of the adipocyte adding to the insulin resistance feedback loop. Once the glucose runs out, and the adipocyte starts to shrink, the inflammation will also stop.

Fatty liver disease also causes the production of inflammatory cytokines. As much as 5% of the cells within the liver are called Kupffer cells, essentially liver-specific macrophages (the immune cells that gather up garbage, and help sound the alarm when something foreign is detected). The stress placed on a fatty liver may trigger the Kupffer cells to produce cytokines, and heighten insulin resistance. And as will be discussed later, fatty liver is caused exclusively by excess dietary carbohydrates (including alcohol). Dietary fats bypass the liver entirely.

Summary: Inflammation is triggered by several processes, and usually elevates blood glucose levels, to make more glucose available to the immune system. When inflammation results from chronic conditions, this contributes to diabetes.

Development of the Feedback Loop

We've reviewed several mechanisms and causes of insulin resistance, and yet all of them stem from the innate programming within cells, leading us to believe it is a natural response. Insulin resistance in the simplest case redirects glucose to the liver, for conversion to fat. In the case of inflammation, it re-works the body's metabolism to fight an infection, rather than exercise or build fat reserves.

At this point, the alert reader may say, "Okay, that sounds like a coherent story, but for one element: Why does the natural process spin out of control and cause diabetes, typically in middle age. Why can a young person eat too many carbs for so many years, and get away with it, but come our mid forties, we start coming down with diabetes? There are several factors that probably play a role, so let's review them.

The muscles of young people are able to churn through a giant bolus of glucose, and their liver has a high capacity to convert it to fat. Eventually, however, we transition from a sugar high to a *sugar coma*, as it is sometimes called. I recall experiencing that by around age 30, when I attended seminars where coffee and cookies were served. Eating a couple of cookies, then sitting down and listening, I found myself falling asleep, even on those occasions when I found the subject matter very interesting. In retrospect, that surely represented the first indications that insulin resistance had started. I could still function well athletically, and burn off excess calories, so my blood glucose was stable. But had I cut out all carbs for six months or so, to simulate a long winter without access to carbs, I now believe I could have reset my system to factory specifications. Likewise, those who fast periodically may be able to reset their system, and eliminate insulin resistance. Competitive athletes, and others who regularly deplete their glycogen reserves probably do not experience insulin resistance in the muscles, which are regularly hungry to replenish their reserves.

As the rates of sugar consumption and obesity among the young have exploded, the sugar high is increasingly rare. It is said that obese children never experience a sugar high. Younger and younger are the reports of insulin resistance, and even type II diabetes. This tells us that age is not the sole factor that triggers the development of diabetes. Age simply lowers the threshold for insulin resistance to spin out of control.

But there are undeniably physiological changes that occur in our early forties. Many of us had twitchy legs when we were young. While sitting, muscles would contract, and the leg would bounce rhythmically. That burned excess energy. How many of us are like that at 50? We are no longer capable of burning excess energy like we once were. So if the muscles can't burn as much energy, they won't be taking up as much fuel, right? The muscles take up less glucose, which accentuates insulin resistance. Next are the mitochondria of the liver. Before, they could burn off a good amount of alcohol and fructose, simply with their elevated metabolic rate. Now, that capacity is diminished, so the liver converts the excess calories to fat. Once the fat builds up, and circulates freely, muscle insulin resistance is increased. Note that this is the only circumstance under which fat and glucose both circulate in high amounts, for an extended period of time. Type II Diabetics, with astronomically high insulin levels, quickly absorb dietary fat into adipocytes.

Insulin levels climb ever higher, to combat the elevated glucose levels, and for some period of time, the liver continues to convert the excess glucose to fat. As long as glucose intake continues to be in excess, however, the loop is continuously amplified. More fat from the liver causes more insulin resistance, causes higher glucose in the blood, causes higher insulin secretion. Eventually, when enough fat builds up in the liver, it triggers inflammation, and insulin resistance in the liver. At this point, the muscles and liver cannot respond to insulin as much as they used to, and the excess glucose consumed in the diet has nowhere to go. It now stays in the blood, and the person is diabetic. How long it takes to reach this stage depends on many factors, including age, genetics, and dietary specifics. But the fuel that keeps the loop going is chronic carbohydrate intake, in excess of what can be metabolized before the next meal. If the fuel is cut off, the feedback loop literally runs out of fuel, like a hurricane after it makes landfall. In a short time, glycogen stores are depleted, insulin resistance drops, blood glucose drops, and equilibrium is restored.

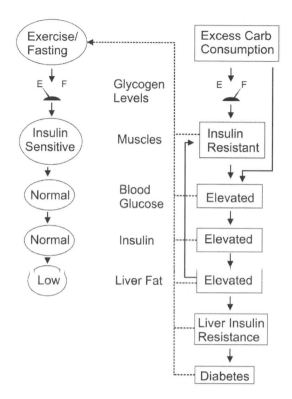

The Feedback Loop: Excess carb consumption, after glycogen reserves are full, initiates insulin resistance. Blood glucose rises, insulin levels rise, and the liver processes the excess, as long as it is able to keep up. In the face of continued excess carb consumption, blood glucose keeps spiking, and insulin levels rise to meet those elevated levels. Cells become more resistant to insulin, to avoid toxic levels of glucose inside them. The liver initially converts the excess to fat, but eventually can't keep up. Fat buildup in the liver spills into the blood, further heightening insulin resistance. Once the liver starts to become inflamed, it starts to become insulin resistant. At that point, the person is diabetic, because there's nowhere for the excess glucose to go. However, if excess glucose intake is stopped, it becomes possible to reverse the whole process, deplete glycogen reserves, and restore insulin sensitivity (dotted line). That is how the feedback loop is broken: Deny it the fuel that keeps it going.

Summary: Insulin resistance evolves from muscles, to liver fat, to inflammation. Along the way, insulin levels keep rising, until they can no longer rise enough to keep up with increasing insulin resistance, and diabetes results. But cutting off the fuel of insulin resistance, namely glucose, can break the loop.

Chapter 2: The Problem With Carbohydrates

Let food be thy medicine and medicine be thy food. ~ Hippocrates

Sugars and Carbohydrates

All biological systems ultimately get their energy from the sun. The sun shines on plants, which use its energy to split molecules of water, and combine it with carbon dioxide, to produce glucose. Plants use glucose for energy, and structure. A large amount of their glucose gets joined together in long, stable chains, to form cellulose. Cellulose makes up all the hard, unappetizing parts of the plant. We refer to cellulose as insoluble fiber. It passes through us without digestion, so to us, it has no calories. Plants can also store starch in their roots, or in grains, which like cellulose is composed of glucose units, but joined together in a way that is easily reversed. To us, cooked potatoes have vastly more calories than an equal weight of hay, and yet they're very similar, chemically. Herbivores have bacteria in their guts that break down cellulose, liberating glucose. And those animals store considerable amounts of fat. It is not difficult, when from their perspective, they are eating a field green with the equivalent of spaghetti.

A small fraction of the carbohydrate made by plants is converted to sugar, or sucrose. Blossoms contain nectar with sucrose, to lure bees. Many fruits are laden with sucrose. Sugar cane has sucrose rich fluid in its stem, which is refined into the white toxin in your kitchen. The sucrose molecule consists of a single unit of glucose and a single unit of fructose, joined by a weak bond. That bond is broken very quickly in the gut, turning sucrose into an equal mixture of glucose and fructose. It makes no difference where that sucrose comes from. It is identical to every other form of sucrose. *Dehydrated organic cane juice concentrate* is identical to ordinary table sugar. High-fructose corn syrup is an industrially produced mixture of glucose and fructose, in roughly equal proportions. Once in the gut, there is literally no difference between sucrose and high-fructose corn syrup.

In the gut, complex sugars are broken down to simple sugars. Sucrose is converted to a natural equivalent of HFCS, and starches are broken down to units of glucose. It is those single units of glucose or fructose that are absorbed into the blood. Glucose can be utilized by every cell in the body, and a considerable amount can be stored in muscles and liver, as chains of glycogen. Glycogen is easy to break apart, to generate glucose rapidly, when needed. Accumulation of glycogen limits the formation of more glycogen, and in muscles, it inhibits further glucose uptake. We can call that insulin resistance, but we should note that it is highly reversible. Athletes who regularly deplete their glycogen stores can build slightly larger reserves than the majority of us who are largely sedentary. The typical middle aged person, however, comes to the dinner table with mostly full glycogen stores, so most of the carbs consumed at dinner will be rejected by the muscles, sent to the liver, and converted to fat.

In addition to glucose, dietary simple sugars include galactose and fructose. Both are more reactive than glucose, and neither is allowed to circulate freely. Galactose is rapidly converted to glucose, which can be used as fuel by every cell in the body.

When glucose is broken down, it ends up as acetyl-CoA, which can either be burned for energy by the cellular engines, known as the mitochondria, or if the mitochondria are busy with a glut of acetyl-CoA, converted to fat. Fructose, on the other hand, cannot be stored by the liver, or taken up in significant quantity by any organ other than the liver. It must be quickly burned as fuel, or converted to fat. All the fructose in a bottle of sweet soda pop or juice goes straight to the liver, and all of it directly to the mitochondria in the liver. That is too much, too fast. Inevitably, most of it is converted to fat. And because the liver's mitochondria are at capacity using up the acetyl-CoA from fructose, any excess glucose is also converted to fat.

The following table shows what happens when one hundred calories of glucose are consumed, versus one hundred calories of sucrose, or HFCS:

100 calories consumed	Body	Liver
Glucose	80	20
Sucrose/HFCS		
Fructose	0	50
Glucose	40	10

The calories going to the liver are sixty from sucrose/HFCS, versus twenty from glucose. This initiates fat synthesis, and creates a traffic jam at the liver. Glucose builds up in the blood, more insulin is secreted, and eventually we get the start of insulin resistance. After that, much more glucose is diverted to the liver, as insulin resistance cuts off other destinations for glucose.

Summary: Glucose is the primary fuel made by plants, using sunlight as energy. It can be incorporated into long chains, for storage or structure. Glucose can be used as fuel by any cell in the body, whereas fructose can only be used by the liver, and cannot be stored. If the liver has more fuel than it can use at one time, it turns the excess into fat.

Sugars Are Toxic, in Blood *AND* in Cells

Glucose and the other simple sugars can exist in two forms. In one form, glucose is a cyclic molecule, where the reactive groups are blocked. Most glucose exists in this more stable form, and when incorporated into chains such as glycogen, all glucose is cyclic. But when dissolved in water, approximately 3% of single glucose units exist in a linear form, where a reactive aldehyde group is exposed. This property, which makes glucose a ready source of energy, also predisposes it to react with proteins all over the body, in places where it does no good, and can cause considerable harm.

Glucose

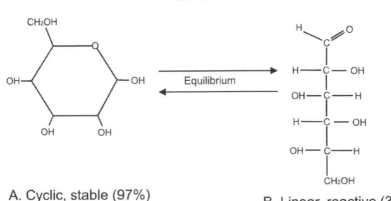

A. Cyclic, stable (97%)
B. Linear, reactive (3%)

Have you ever wondered what makes toast turn brown? Or how you get that crispy, light brown surface on French fries or hash browns? It is from the reaction of glucose with other molecules, stimulated by the heat applied to them. Glucose can react with proteins, lipids, and even nucleic acids (yes, even DNA). The slow, spontaneous reaction of glucose with other molecules is called *glycation*. Heat accelerates the reaction, such as by cooking, but no enzymes are required for the process to happen.

The reactivity of glucose forms the basis for the HbA1C test. It measures the percentage (or millimolar concentration) of hemoglobin molecules that have been glycated at the first amino acid position. Everybody has some A1C, and the amount is proportional to the average glucose concentration in the blood over about the previous three months, the lifespan of hemoglobin. Technically, this is an example of the damage glucose inflicts on proteins. The function of hemoglobin is not harmed by glycation, so measuring it is merely a convenient way to estimate the damage glucose has done elsewhere. But the function of many other proteins is impaired by reaction with glucose or fructose. And in the extreme, glycated proteins can form a cross-linked tangle, leading to an inflammatory response.

Fructose is much more reactive than glucose. Glucose is the least reactive simple sugar, and the least toxic. Fructose glycates hemoglobin at several places, at an effective rate ten times that of glucose. So like any toxin, it is important to remove it from circulation as fast as possible. This task falls on the liver, and the price to be paid is that the mitochondria in the liver are overloaded for some time, as fructose is metabolized. Damage to the circulatory system is normally attributed to glucose itself, as fructose gets absorbed by the liver at high efficiency. But as no test measures blood fructose levels, we don't know how much toxicity it causes when the liver is overloaded, and some fructose circulates freely.

Glucose in the blood comes into constant contact with the extra-cellular matrix, the mesh of scaffold proteins that anchor cells throughout the body, particularly those of the vascular endothelium. The vascular endothelium comprises the network of small blood vessels, known as the *microvasculature*, and lines the inside of veins and arteries. Glycation of the extra-cellular matrix is thought to weaken its ability to support vascular endothelial cells. We'll return to this question when we discuss why diabetes predisposes to heart disease. Everyone has glucose in their blood, but at healthy levels, the matrix is replaced quickly enough that glycation does not lead to blood vessel damage. But elevated glucose levels, over a long period of time, will cause damage to the microvasculature. It's glucose concentration (presumably plus any fructose times ten), multiplied by the duration of that elevated glucose, that determines the extent of the damage.

If the only problem was sugar in the blood, then we would expect it to be solved by removing sugars from blood. Coax cells to take up glucose, and forget about it. Alas, this is medicine's first fatal error. Like skin, the vascular endothelium covers the tissue beneath. And the cells of the vascular endothelium die if faced with excessive intra-cellular glucose, which contributes to arterial wounding and heart disease. But what about the liver, where glucose goes for storage as glycogen, or conversion to fat? It may be less sensitive than vascular endothelium, but all cells have a mechanism in place to limit the concentration of free intra-cellular glucose. If there's too much, they refuse more. We call that insulin resistance, and consider it an obstacle to be overcome. But it should instead be viewed as a cellular defense mechanism. Defense from what?

Glycation happens inside cells as much as in circulation. And with each glycation event, reactive oxygen species are released. Cells have limited capacity to neutralize reactive oxygen. Once exhausted, the cell dies in an oxidative cascade that threatens to spread to other cells, and unleashes an inflammatory response that can stress the whole organ. Is that what we want to happen to the liver? Because that's what our current strategy of force-feeding glucose to the liver is doing. Later, I'll link liver dysfunction to the development of heart disease.

Finally, there is the problem of cancer. Diabetics have much higher cancer rates than those with healthy glucose metabolism. One old question was whether it was the elevated glucose itself that was responsible, or the elevated insulin levels that are characteristic of insulin resistant (type II) diabetes. For an answer to that question, we can compare the rates of cancer for type I diabetics, who only have what insulin they inject, which tends to be low. Their cancer rates are lower than those for type II diabetics, but still higher than healthy individuals. Since type I diabetics are exposed to high blood glucose, but not to high insulin levels, while type II diabetics are exposed to both, three gradations of cancer risk suggest that both insulin and glucose factor into the elevated cancer rates.

	Glucose	Insulin	Cancer Risk
Normal Glucose	Normal	Low	Low
Type I Diabetes	High	Low	Intermediate
Type II Diabetes	High	Very High	High

Is it the reactivity of glucose that causes cancer? It can even react with DNA, after all. This is where things get complicated. Glucose levels inside the cells of untreated diabetics are not normally elevated. It's *blood* glucose that is elevated. Accordingly, in an untreated type II diabetic, we would not expect there to be any diabetes-related DNA damage. When treated, however, we can no longer make that generalization, because the objective of type II diabetes treatment is to shove more glucose into cells than they are willing to take. The defensive response is subverted, and DNA damage becomes a possibility.

A second mechanism has been known for nearly a century, and is called the Warburg Effect. In 1924, biochemist Otto Warburg observed that cancer cells obtained their energy from glycolysis, or the fermentation of glucose, without oxidative respiration. This was true even when oxygen was in ready supply. This is glaringly obvious when growing cultures of cancer cells in the laboratory. The cell growth medium contains a dye that changes color with a change in pH. One can see with a single glance if the medium has turned acidic. And the more aggressive the cancer cells, the more acidic they turn the medium, from the accumulation of lactic acid. The cells are fermenting glucose, rather than oxidizing it. In modern times, science has learned that solid tumors are not adequately permeated by blood vessels to allow oxygen delivery, or for that matter, delivery of effective doses of chemotherapeutic agents.

Fermentation is a far less efficient way to produce energy than oxidative respiration, and therefore requires vastly more glucose to meet the cell's energy needs. So given cancer cells' reliance on glycolysis, elevated glucose in the blood provides those cancer cells with the extra fuel they require, and without which they would likely not survive. Modern research has also shown that cancer cells have far fewer mitochondria than normal cells, and those they have are defective. This may not be a surprise, given their oxygen-poor environment. But mitochondria have a second job in the cell, which is no less important than making energy. When a cell goes bad, such as becoming a cancer cell, functioning mitochondria send a self-destruct signal to the rest of the cell. The tightly choreographed process is called *apoptosis*, and is often described as *programmed cell death*. Being orderly, it does not cause inflammation. It might be that cancer cells' mitochondria *have to be* defective, or the cancer would never arise and survive.

Given all the dangers of elevated blood glucose, it is imperative to bring it under control. But the manner in which it is brought under control is the subject at hand. Medical strategies that rely on simply stuffing ever more glucose into cells, thinking the problem is behind them, simply transfer the toxicity into cells, where the damage can potentially be more severe. When ranked as independent risk factors for heart disease, diabetes ranks very high as a risk factor, whereas elevated blood glucose does not (BMJ 1997, 315:722). How does one separate the two? Because after diagnosis of type II diabetes, drugs stuff glucose into cells, and reduce its concentration in the blood. Glucose looks controlled, yet heart disease risk is not reduced. We'll discuss the links between diabetes and heart disease later, but one of the contributors is likely liver stress, caused by forced glucose overload.

Summary: Glucose and fructose are toxic. They are chemically reactive, and will react with the scaffold that holds blood vessels together, as well as anything they contact inside cells. Cellular toxicity may be even greater than blood toxicity, when diabetes drugs shove ever more glucose into cells. Cancer cells need large amounts of glucose, and may not survive without it.

Glucose Transport

Glucose crosses cell membranes too slowly to be of any use, if left to passive diffusion. Instead, a specialized type of protein, called a *glucose transporter*, shuttles the glucose molecule into a cell. Ignoring the minor players (of which there are many), let's focus on the four major glucose transporters throughout the body. They carry the prefix *GLUT* and a number between one and four.

	Location	Function
GLUT1	All cells, low amounts	Uptake of glucose, vitamin C
GLUT2	Liver, kidney	Reversibly shuttles glucose in and out of cells
GLUT3	Brain, some cancers	Very high activity, always on
GLUT4	Liver, muscle, fat cells	Regulated uptake of glucose

The first point is that of the four principal glucose transporters, GLUT1, GLUT2, and GLUT3 are entirely independent of insulin. Only GLUT4 is regulated by insulin, allowing for regulation of glucose uptake by muscle, liver, and fat cells. And wherever there's regulation, it creates the possibility of turning the whole thing off.

GLUT4 hides inside the cell when not needed, and is effectively turned *off*. But when summoned by insulin action, GLUT4 moves to the cell surface, where it imports very large quantities of glucose into cells. A total of 70% of all glucose taken up from the blood after a carb-rich meal is by the action of GLUT4, due to the large quantity of GLUT4 in cells that are targets for insulin. When insulin resistance develops, GLUT4 fails to move to the cell surface in response to insulin, and excess glucose is not taken up from the blood. Accordingly, regulation of GLUT4 movement to the cell surface has always been the focus of attention in diabetes drug development. But rather than seeing this as a technical obstacle, we should focus on the reason why GLUT4 is the insulin-responsive transporter, allowing for the possibility of insulin resistance. GLUT3, for instance, is a very powerful glucose transporter that is independent of insulin. It could have been used in liver and muscle, if the only objective were clearing glucose from the blood. But GLUT3 is generally restricted to the brain, where it delivers a steady stream of glucose, without any interference.

While GLUT4 is the only regulated glucose transporter, insulin is far from the only stimulus that can make it move to the cell surface. The mechanical action of muscle contraction directly shuttles GLUT4 to the cell surface. This is certainly not an accident, since muscle contraction presumes the need for fuel. This is independent of insulin, and is fully intact in all diabetics. And one other stimulus can trigger GLUT4 movement to the cell surface: Cell starvation. Cells that run low on energy have a program to quickly get that energy when they need it. It consists of a system that senses the accumulation of a metabolite (AMP) that forms when energy stores in the form of adenosine triphosphate (ATP) drop to low levels.

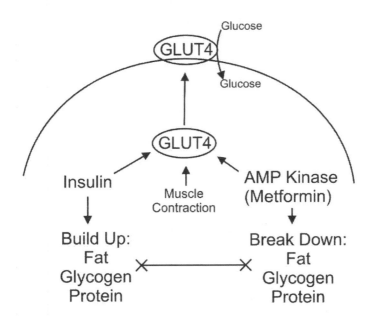

The response to low energy levels involves a protein called AMP kinase, which sounds the alarm all over the cell. First, GLUT4 is shuttled to the cell surface, to get fuel. Second, glucose stored in the form of glycogen is liberated, for immediate use as fuel. Third, fats and proteins are broken down, to provide additional sources of fuel. In summary, insulin, muscle contraction, and AMP Kinase all cause GLUT4 to move to the surface, and take up glucose (reviewed by Huang and Czech, Cell Metabolism 5:237-252, 2007). At first glance, they all seem to reinforce each other. But looking deeper,

AMP Kinase and insulin have opposite effects *inside* the cell. The starvation response is trying to break things down, to obtain fuel, while the insulin response is giving the opposite instruction, because there's an excess of fuel. AMP Kinase is significant in medicine, because it is the target of the diabetes drug metformin.

What happens when the starvation response is active, and the person eats a meal rich in glucose? The answer: Insulin wins, if we're talking about a young, healthy individual. The blood glucose spike will activate the insulin response, cellular energy levels rise, and AMP kinase will go quiet. But in the meantime, the insulin response effectively says to the starvation response, "Shut up, your food is coming," by directly shutting off AMP kinase. There is no point breaking down the body's tissues, when more fuel is only moments away. This is another useful reminder that everything biological is tightly regulated, and every contradiction is accounted for, and integrated.

Summary: Glucose doesn't simply diffuse into cells. It needs to be shuttled in. There are many ways for cells to achieve this, and get their glucose. Insulin-stimulated glucose uptake is only one of many, and is only relevant in muscles, liver, and fat cells. Even the muscles and liver do not strictly need insulin to get their glucose. Insulin works opposite the cell starvation response, but both cause glucose uptake. Diabetes drugs often stimulate both, in combination, regardless that most of their effects are contradictory.

What Cells Do With Glucose

Insulin resistance can be seen as the refusal by cells to respond to the insulin signal. We attempt to override that refusal, in order to remove more glucose from the blood. But what are cells supposed to do with all the glucose we're forcing them to take up? Here are the various options.

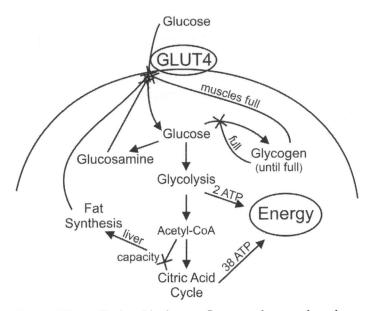

Figure: What cells do with glucose. Some can be stored as glycogen, but once muscles are full, they block more glucose uptake. Some can be burned for immediate energy, but that has limits. Excess acetyl-CoA is used to make fat in the liver, which accumulates and blocks glucose uptake. Finally, some is shuttled off to make glucosamine, which is a sensor that keeps cellular glucose levels under control, by blocking more glucose uptake. Overuse of any of these three natural processes builds insulin resistance.

1. Burn the Glucose

The most obvious use for glucose is to burn it, to generate energy. Glucose is after all suitable for use by every cell in the body. And there are two ways in which glucose can be used to make energy: Fermentation, and respiration. The start of the two pathways looks the same, and respiration simply takes the process further. Fermentation breaks glucose down to smaller molecules, and two units of energy are produced (energy units being molecules of ATP - the cellular energy store). This breakdown of glucose is called *glycolysis*, and it occurs without the input of any oxygen, which is why it is also called *anaerobic*. An intermediate end product of the pathway is pyruvate. Pyruvate can be converted to acetyl-CoA, which enters the citric acid cycle. The citric acid cycle burns fuel using oxygen (and is called aerobic) and yields 38 energy units per glucose molecule (versus 2 units for the anaerobic pathway).

If too much pyruvate accumulates, it is converted to lactic acid. Quick bursts of speed or power by athletes generates considerable lactic acid in their muscles, and can cause cramping. A period of rest is needed for the muscles to catch up, and clear the lactic acid. Lactic acid is then shuttled to the liver, and used to regenerate glucose. The process is inefficient, and consumes significant calories. The appearance of new glucose is slow, and in most cases does not appreciably raise blood glucose levels. It seems, then, that quick bursts of exercise are a very effective way to reduce excess blood glucose. That is, for young athletes, not middle aged sedentary people. The difference is in the makeup of our muscles. Young athletes have a lot of fast-twitch muscle, which can ferment a lot of glucose in a hurry. As we age, the composition of our muscles changes to slow-twitch, which use oxygen to generate energy much more efficiently, but more slowly. Thus, by the age at which type II diabetes is a serious concern, fast twitch muscle is no longer an efficient glucose sink. The change in muscle composition is likely one factor that determines why type II diabetes usually strikes in middle age.

A second factor that affects our ability to metabolize glucose, or any other fuel, is the health of our mitochondria, the cellular energy factories. Sedentary people tend to have old mitochondria, inefficient at their work. In some cases, mitochondria are gummed up by trans fats, and other unnatural fuels they cannot quite finish off. In other cases, it is simply disuse that is responsible. Exercise is an excellent stimulator of mitochondrial turnover, replacing old ones with new, healthy ones. But even then, our mitochondria in middle age are simply not as efficient as those of young people. Think how rare it is for any professional athlete to compete past their early forties.

But even for those who exercise regularly, and strenuously, it is exceedingly difficult to exercise enough to offset excessive glucose consumption. One estimate I found was that it takes a walk of 2.5 miles (4 km) to burn the sugar in one candy bar, or can of sweet soda pop. If a plate of pasta preceded it, then it becomes essentially impossible. The bottom line is that almost nobody over the age of fifty, and that includes very active, fit people, can consistently burn up all the glucose consumed in the standard American diet. The result is an accumulation of acetyl-CoA in the liver, over and above amounts that can be used in the citric acid cycle.

2. Store Glucose as Glycogen

Insulin stimulates the synthesis of glycogen, which is a chain of glucose molecules, joined end to end. It is a simple reaction, and is quickly reversed, so a large amount of glucose can be made available on demand. While bound up as glycogen, glucose remains nonreactive, and non-toxic. The liver can store on the order of 100 grams of glycogen, and the muscles, about 400 grams. Elite athletes can store a little more. In aggregate, it represents more than one pound of glucose. Of course, by middle-age, the capacity of muscles to store glycogen has decreased, especially if the person is mostly sedentary. After all, if muscle composition in middle age is no longer optimized for quick bursts of energy fueled by glycolysis, there is little point storing as much glycogen. One way to think of it is that the body can store something like one day's recommended total carbohydrate intake, if one follows the dietary guidelines.

The question is what happens the next day, and the day after that. Unless the stored glycogen is depleted before eating again, there is decreased capacity to store it. Glycogen storage is regulated by cells, and increased glycogen content inhibits insulin-stimulated glucose uptake.

Some will point out that glycogen storage disorders such as von Gierke's disease result in an enormous buildup of glycogen in the liver, suggesting that glycogen accumulation is not limited. The problem with that reasoning is that athletes who might benefit from storing more glycogen cannot remotely approach those quantities, even with extensive training and adaptation. As long as the system is in equilibrium, glycogen storage is effectively limited.

When someone has been depleted of glycogen, for instance after a long fast, and is then fed carbohydrates, the liver is the first organ to take up its share of glucose, to be stored as glycogen. While fasting, free fatty acids support the energy needs of muscles, and they are effectively insulin resistant. Then after a meal, the insulin signal immediately blocks the release of more fatty acids from adipocytes. Those in circulation are used up, and by the time the liver has its fill of glycogen, the muscles are ready to take up glucose, and build glycogen reserves. At modest amounts of glucose, the system remains in equilibrium, especially if the person engages in periodic fasting and regular exercise.

But if carbohydrate consumption continues in excess, the body runs out of cells willing to take up the excess glucose. What follows is a traffic jam of glucose molecules in the blood, waiting to get inside a cell that will accommodate them. Initially, this is the liver, but it can only take up glucose as quickly as it can convert the excess it already has into fat.

3. Convert Glucose to Fat

When the liver has reached its glycogen storage capacity, and glucose continues to be in excess, more acetyl-CoA accumulates than can be used in the citric acid cycle. Accumulation of acetyl-CoA, especially when insulin signaling is active, informs the liver to convert the excess to fat. And if there is a chronic excess of glucose, then fat production will continue without pause. In principle, this is a practical solution, because the body can store much more fat than it can glycogen. We next need to examine what happens to the fat produced by the liver.

The preferred destination for fat is the sub-cutaneous adipocytes. I know most of us would rather have fewer of them, or at least for the ones we have to be smaller, but that is the best place for it. A certain amount of fat is stored inside the abdomen, and is called visceral fat. Its accumulation is said to be associated with diabetes and its complications. It is also known to make numerous cytokines, increasing insulin resistance, high blood pressure, and inflammation. And it is considered a high risk factor for heart disease. Fortunately, visceral fat is the easiest to lose, suggesting it is but an overflow valve, for when the liver produces excessive amounts of fat in a short time, and cannot export it all to the subcutaneous fat reserves.

Finally, when the system is utterly swamped, droplets of fat accumulate in the liver, causing fatty liver disease, which raises the risk of heart disease, and can lead to liver failure. Heavy alcohol consumption also causes fatty liver. Only when someone is a non-drinker, or close to it, is it referred to as non-alcoholic fatty liver disease, and are dietary remedies imposed. When the patient drinks more than a token amount, it is considered alcohol-induced. But pediatric endocrinologist Robert Lustig, who treats obese children and conducts research on the topic, insists they are fundamentally the same disease. In both cases, the liver is chronically overloaded by a carbohydrate, converts it to fat, and if it is too much, too quickly, it accumulates in the liver. Lustig points out that fructose, much like alcohol, is only metabolized by the liver, and in amounts above what can be burned by the liver's mitochondria, is converted to fat. The effects of alcohol and fructose are presumably additive. So now you know why that strawberry daiquiri, containing both sugar and alcohol, is so fattening.

In summary, the liver converts excess carbohydrates to fat, and over short intervals, it is probably normal. It is when it becomes chronic that complications arise, and the health consequences become progressively worse. And if the liver is working flat out, there is likely to be a backlog of glucose, waiting in the bloodstream, for its turn to enter the liver.

4. Convert Glucose to Glucosamine

There is one final alternative for what the cell can do with all that glucose. Between 2% and 5% of intracellular glucose is diverted from the regular energy-producing pathways, and is converted to glucosamine. Given the low percentage of glucose going down this pathway, it is not a significant *sink* of glucose, but instead serves as a metabolic regulatory mechanism.

Very precise enzymes attach glucosamine to as many as 4,000 different proteins within the cell, in a process called glycosylation (unlike glycation, which happens without any enzymatic action). Glycosylation is reversible, and when it happens in short, transient bursts, is essential for the protection of heart cells from metabolic stress (Fulop et al., Am J Physiol Heart Circ Physiol. 292: 2227-2236, 2007).

Many of the proteins involved in moving GLUT4 to the cell surface, and stimulating glucose uptake, are targets for glycosylation. In every case, glycosylation impairs, or blocks, the function of that protein. Or it stimulates antagonists of glucose uptake. The net effect is that excess glucose inside the cell impairs the uptake of more glucose; a textbook case of negative feedback.

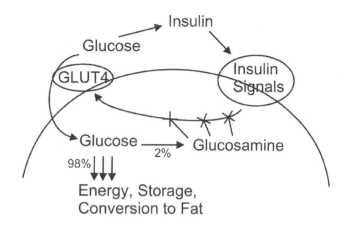

The glucosamine pathway serves to protect cells from oxidative stress induced by excess glucose. Every time a glucose molecule reacts with another molecule, it gives rise to reactive oxygen. In the blood, quite a bit of oxygen can be mopped up, as it has to be, given the high oxygen content of blood. But inside cells, reactive oxygen is much more problematic. If it gets into the cell membrane, it can literally cause a chain reaction, and tear the cell apart. If it reacts with DNA, mutations and/or cancer can result. Mitochondria, that regularly generate reactive oxygen, are paired with structures known as peroxisomes, whose only job is to detoxify oxygen. If the oxygen is generated anywhere else in the cell, the only remaining defense is glutathione, a sulfur compound maintained by cells to mop up oxygen. But it can easily be depleted, and oxidative damage can result. That is why this mechanism exists, to place very tight control on glucose concentrations inside the cell.

As always, the problem is compounded when the glucose elevation is chronic. Then, glycosylation moves beyond directly affecting the function of proteins involved in regulation of glucose uptake, and induces epigenetic changes on genes, making insulin resistance more stable, over a longer period of time. And chronic glycosylation is thought to be directly toxic to the vascular endothelial smooth muscle cells that comprise the microvasculature. So it contributes directly to the vascular degradation responsible for the complications of diabetes.

When excess glucose is chronic, glycosylation is a cellular protective response that greatly *increases* insulin resistance. In an early draft of this book, I said glycosylation *worsens* insulin resistance. I initially held the mainstream medical idea of insulin resistance as something to be forcibly overcome. Publications characterizing glycosylation always include speculation about how it might be artificially subverted, as a diabetes treatment strategy. When the only objective is reducing blood glucose, this is the kind of toxic idea it breeds.

To conclude, insulin resistance should not be considered a *problem* to be overcome, but as an evolution of several processes, which in the beginning serve to make maximal use of available energy, and at advanced stages, to limit glucose toxicity imposed on the cells of the body. As bad as excessive glucose in the blood is, excessive glucose in cells is worse. There is a class of diabetes drugs (reviewed in Appendix II) called the *glitazones*, that overcome the insulin resistance of the liver, by changing gene expression patterns. The first ones were withdrawn from market for liver toxicity, and new ones are being closely watched over the same concerns. In other cases, toxicity would probably be mistaken for a common complication of diabetes, and would not be reported as a recognized side-effect of any treatment strategy.

Summary: Cells can burn glucose, but only at a certain rate. Muscle and liver can store more, but that too is limited. The liver can convert glucose to fat, but even that is limited. When glucose intake exceeds all of the above, high blood glucose is the inevitable result. Lastly, cells have a built-in protection mechanism, to ensure they don't get too much glucose inside them. This avoids toxicity. Some diabetes drugs try to override that protection mechanism, and some have been withdrawn from market, due to liver toxicity.

The Problem of Metformin

Metformin is typically the first drug prescribed to a type II diabetic. It used to be marketed under the name *Glucophage,* which means *glucose-eater.* And that's what it does. It makes cells eat glucose, to remove it from the blood. As introduced above, it directly stimulates AMP Kinase, which is supposed to sense cell starvation. Except that metformin stimulates AMP Kinase even when the cell is not starved, but is swimming in excess glucose.

One of the problems faced by type II diabetics is fatty liver disease. The liver converts excess carbs to fat too quickly, and some of it builds up as droplets in the liver. Eventually, the fat causes inflammation of the liver, and markers of liver stress appear in the blood. One treatment that seems effective is metformin. This may seem a paradox, at first. Fatty liver is caused by a chronic excess of carbs taken up by the liver, yet it is cured by an agent that makes the liver take up even more. The answer is clear once we realize that glucose uptake is not the relevant factor.

It's true that both insulin and metformin cause glucose uptake, but beyond that, their effects are opposite. Insulin stimulates fat production, while metformin blocks it. Insulin stimulates glycogen synthesis, while metformin also blocks and reverses that. Remember that metformin activates the cell starvation response, which thinks the cell needs energy on an emergency basis. You don't store glucose as glycogen, or convert it to fat for long-term storage when you're starving. You use it immediately, for energy right now. Blocking fat production by the liver will give the liver a chance to clear excess fat, which is probably why metformin is effective against fatty liver disease. But what is the liver supposed to do with the excess glucose it is forced to take up, under the false signal that it is starving? It can't store it. Some gets converted to glucosamine, which accentuates insulin resistance, but metformin bypasses insulin resistance, and continues to stuff the cell with more glucose.

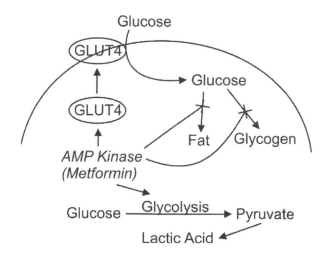

The cell starvation response also stimulates glucose fermentation, or glycolysis, to generate energy immediately. So a lot of excess glucose is fermented, and an excess of pyruvate accumulates. Ideally, pyruvate is converted to acetyl-CoA, and enters the citric acid cycle, to make a lot of energy. But the mitochondria can only work so fast. Eventually, there is more fuel than the cell can use. That backs things up, and excess pyruvate is converted to lactic acid. Metformin can occasionally cause a recognized acute condition called *lactic acidosis* in the liver. You could call that lactic acid poisoning. But what happens at sub-acute levels? A diabetic can be on metformin for twenty years or more, and the drug is not giving cells a good option for what to do with all that glucose, other than turning it into lactic acid.

One of the more dubious pieces of medical advice I've seen said that diabetes causes chronic fatigue syndrome/fibromyalgia because cells can't get enough glucose, and are tired. But as discussed here, cells don't need insulin to get glucose from blood. Insulin is not even used when energy is needed. It is only used when energy is in surplus, and needs to be stored. Instead, why don't we ask whether the buildup of lactic acid is responsible for fibromyalgia? There are plenty of reports linking the two, and the widespread use of metformin explains the link perfectly.

Given that there are two alternative, and largely contradictory ways to cause GLUT4 movement to the cell surface, which one should be used to treat diabetes? The cell starvation response, or a boosted insulin response? Experienced clinicians already know the answer. Since clearing glucose from circulation is medicine's only consideration, both are used, often in combination. Yet most of the instructions being given to cells by the combination of metformin and insulin are mutually contradictory. Current practice disregards this fact, and only concerns itself with the blood glucose number, while maintaining a high carbohydrate diet.

The cells of a young, healthy person will obey the insulin signal, and shut off the AMP kinase signal. They will then store some amount of glucose as glycogen. But that person is not given metformin. The person prescribed metformin is insulin resistant, so a conflict of signals has to be resolved. How it is resolved depends on the degree of insulin resistance, the dosage of each drug, and the timing of administration. The greater the insulin resistance, and the higher the dose of metformin, the more the balance will favor the cell starvation response, and lactic acid buildup. Elevated glucose in liver cells causes oxidative damage, stress on the liver, and the risk of heart disease may be increased. If this treatment continues for over twenty years, as it often does in the course of diabetes, could this contribute to the high risk of heart disease among diabetics? It's not on the list of known side-effects for metformin, but let's not discount the idea. It could be hiding in plain sight; ignored because diabetes itself is considered the cause of heart disease.

There's another lesson in the observation that an intact insulin response shuts off the cell starvation response. Type I diabetics exhibit the symptoms of starvation, in addition to high blood glucose. Type II diabetics, by contrast, are overweight. The difference between them? Insulin. Type I diabetics have only what they inject, where type II diabetics have a chronic excess. We'll re-visit this several times.

Summary: Metformin forces cells to take up glucose, as though the cell were starving. Even when it's over-stuffed with glucose. Metformin also prohibits cells from storing glucose, or converting it to fat. Glucose can only be burned so fast. What options are left? Intracellular glucose is toxic, so this is a concern.

Insulin: The Signal to Fatten Up

If the only function of insulin was to stimulate glucose uptake, then that is all it would do. And if insulin was essential for cells to acquire sufficient energy, then those cells would starve without insulin. But neither of those is true.

We previously discussed how cells have several options for how they import glucose from the blood. Further, the liver and muscles are never in danger of starving from a lack of glucose, even in type I diabetics with no insulin at all. The only cell type that seems to starve in type I diabetes is the adipocyte. This provides an important clue to the true function of insulin.

A second clue is obvious from what happens when type I diabetics repeatedly inject themselves with insulin in the same spot. Over time, fat cells build up exactly where the person injects, and create a visible bulge of fat. Simply put, insulin appears to be a stimulator of fat storage.

At low glucose levels, or with intense exercise, little insulin is needed, and it serves to keep the system in equilibrium. What is of greater interest is what happens when glucose intake is chronically high. Since muscles do not synthesize fat, what do they do with excess glucose, once they max out their glycogen reserves? The answer: They refuse it. This creates flexibility in the metabolic response to glucose consumption. More insulin is secreted, and glucose is sent to the liver, and fat cells, to make and store fat.

Free fatty acids are made by the liver, when it has an excess of carbs or protein, above what the liver's mitochondria can burn as fuel. But fatty acids are the oily part of fat, and with cell membranes being an oily barrier, free fatty acids can cross membranes like they were nothing. As a result, fat cells can't retain and store free fatty acids. To store fat, they need to join free fatty acids to something that cannot cross membranes. That something is glycerol. Glycerol has three hydroxyl groups, that form ester linkages with carboxylic acid groups at the ends of three free fatty acid chains. The whole molecule is called triacylglycerol, or more commonly, triglyceride. Triglycerides are what make up fat, as we know it.

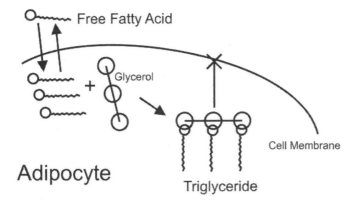

Triglycerides are transported from the liver to fat cells in lipoprotein vesicles, which have a membrane like cells do. Fats cannot exit the vesicle unless the triglyceride is first broken down to free fatty acids and glycerol. The free fatty acids can then cross out of the vesicle, and enter the adipocyte. Inside that fat cell, the fatty acids must again be joined to glycerol, or they are free to leave the fat cell.

Now, let's look at where fat cells get glycerol. It cannot cross from circulation into the adipocyte. It has to be made, metabolically. And there is one essential precursor, without which glycerol cannot be made: Glucose. Further, while other cells can get their glucose by multiple mechanisms, fat cells seem uniquely dependent on insulin for glucose uptake.

I've already mentioned that type I diabetics have excess glucose in their blood, but their adipocytes are starved of it. Without glucose, fat cells cannot make glycerol, and cannot store fat. Give type I diabetics injections of insulin, and they are able to store fat. This is strong proof that insulin is necessary for the storage of fat And that holds even for people without type I diabetes. Without the action of insulin, fat cells cannot hold on to free fatty acids. Those fatty acids spill into the blood, and are used as fuel by the body. That triggers the same response as the eating of fat, when insulin levels are low: Appetite suppression.

But when insulin levels are high, adipocytes always have plenty of glycerol, will quickly vacuum up all available dietary fat, and will not release any. Type II diabetics, then, will see their dietary fat rapidly stored and cleared from circulation, but they remain insulin resistant. This should put to rest the notion that dietary fat causes insulin resistance.

This broader definition of the role of insulin needs to be borne in mind at all times, especially when drugs are prescribed to diabetics with the intent of boosting the power of the insulin response. On the scale of minutes to hours, they may well achieve the objective of scrubbing the blood of excess glucose. But they always activate all the other responses to insulin, serving the goal of making and storing fat.

If it sounds like I am vilifying insulin, it's partly true. High insulin levels are a big part of the problem in type II diabetes, and raising insulin levels even higher is a bad idea. But insulin is a perfectly good (and necessary) hormone, so long as it is used in moderation. The trick is to only *need* to use it in moderation. And that can be quite a trick, given that this is the *feast hormone*. After all, *feasting* essentially implies a lack of moderation, for a period of time.

Summary: Insulin is a signal that coordinates multiple processes throughout the body, with the objective of turning excess carbohydrates into fat, and storing that fat in fat cells. Taking glucose out of circulation is simply how the insulin response gets its fuel to build fat.

The Other Path

Given that insulin resistance is a natural, programmed response, I'd like to pose a question: If diabetes treatment has as its primary objective the circumvention of natural insulin resistance, what are the anticipated consequences of overriding all of these cellular programs? By the time insulin resistance becomes clinically relevant, when the person is diabetic, the scale of response is well into the cellular self-defense mode. The program to build fat in a seasonal manner may no longer be consistent with the way we live, but the cell's defensive program to reject more glucose in the face of a chronic excess, remains essential. When we force cells to continue to take up glucose against their implied wishes (by virtue of their escalating insulin resistance), we build fat, cause inflammation, and in the process, destroy our cardiovascular health. If it were otherwise, diabetes drugs that stuff glucose into cells would reduce the risk of heart disease. They don't.

To put the current medical paradigm into context, imagine a large, modern city in North America. Its people buy too many things, and throw most of them straight into the trash, sometimes with a delay of a few weeks, or months. The administrators of that city are soon faced with a problem: What to do with all that trash. Attempting to build a landfill in any neighborhood causes immediate protests. Proposals for an incinerator will be met with a reception only slightly less hostile than a nuclear power plant. And so, after exhausting their other options, administrators end up coaxing some poor rural community or third world country to accept their trash, in exchange for cash. Nobody thinks it is a great solution. The solution would be to reduce trash production, if that were possible.

Glucose uptake is really the same problem, but on a cellular scale. We consume far more glucose than we can burn through exercise, so our inbuilt program recognizes it as a chance to build fat reserves, leading to insulin resistance, and over time, with additional factors involved, diabetes. Medicine steps in, recognizes insulin resistance as the only obstacle to getting glucose out of the blood, and treats cells like the poor rural communities, forced to take someone else's trash. We try to purge the blood of excess glucose, and give no thought to where it goes afterwards, and what eventually happens to it. When the consequences come back and poison us in another way, it is considered a separate problem, to be treated with different medical interventions.

The practical outcome of the current paradigm (that the only objective is to remove glucose from circulation) is that knowledge is lost of what proportion of the complications of diabetes are due to too much glucose in the blood, versus too much glucose uptake by cells. We discussed earlier how the microvasculature appears to be harmed by both. And cancer cells are perfectly happy to take up endless quantities of glucose to fuel their anaerobic metabolism, establishing that just because something reduces blood glucose, does not automatically mean it is good. Yet when guided only by the glucose uptake paradigm, we lose sight of the big picture, which could guide us to healthier outcomes.

To regain our bearings, let's return to fundamentals. To state the obvious, medicine should enhance the health of the patient. But since the implications of that statement are vague, Western medical practice tends to use surrogate targets in place of overall health, especially when it can assign numbers. Aiming for a fasting blood glucose level below 100 mg/dl (5.5 mM) is an example of a surrogate. That target arose from valid observations, and a reasonable number was derived that separated those with no diabetic concerns from those who should be concerned. Diagnostically, the number makes perfect sense, and anybody who disagrees would probably only tweak the number. So doesn't it also make sense therapeutically? Yes, if it is a signpost along the way to better health. No, if it is the sole objective, regardless how it is achieved. If blood glucose is reduced by putting it somewhere else, where it can cause more harm, the ends do not justify the means.

When the practitioner loses sight of the big picture of overall health, and focuses only on the surrogate marker, then anything that improves the surrogate is considered a benefit. As we discussed earlier, growing cancer cells gladly take up glucose, and reduce its level in the blood. Likewise, if blood glucose is reduced by force-feeding it to the body's cells, it simply transfers the toxicity from blood to cells. The surrogate marker may show improvement, but the overall health of the individual may worsen. Insulin resistance will increase, pancreatic beta cells will begin to die, and the vascular smooth muscle cells of the microvasculature will deteriorate. The kidneys will retain water, and blood pressure will rise. General inflammation will commence. And the patient becomes vulnerable to heart disease, stroke, kidney failure, gangrene of the extremities, and cancer.

But if we return to seeing the primary objective as enhancing health, and avoiding morbidities, then our approach changes. Instead of treating diabetes as a narrowly defined endocrine problem to be solved by overriding the natural, hard-wired cellular response, we can instead think of it as a nutritional problem. We understand that the primary function of insulin is to initiate a series of anabolic processes (the buildup of glycogen and fat), and one important side-effect is a short-term drop in blood glucose levels. Our objective being overall health, we will also target a fasting blood glucose level of below 100 mg/dl. The only difference is that we see the bigger picture, and allow that picture to steer us to the final goal, rather than considering the surrogate number to be the only objective.

Once we make that change in our thinking, we will no longer think of diabetes in terms of finding the right compartment into which to stuff all that glucose. Instead of trying to reduce it in blood by force-feeding it to cells, we will ask whether it would be better to consume less of it. On the surface, it seems obvious that consuming less glucose should lessen the problems associated with too much glucose. So why is this not standard medical thinking? The truth is, it once was (reviewed by Westman and Vernon, Nutr Metab 2008, 5:10). The authors state that it was forgotten as a viable treatment following the discovery of insulin, metformin, and other drugs. The emphasis of the medical system quickly changed to controlling the surrogate marker of blood glucose with pharmacological agents. Fingers are often pointed at pharmaceutical companies, and their advertising budgets can be difficult to prevail against, but they only provide tools for the medical community to use at its discretion. The fingers are better pointed at the leadership of the medical establishment, for leading the medical community to treat the surrogate marker as the primary objective, and the associated hypertension as a second primary objective, rather than seeing the link between the two, and confronting their common cause.

With a holistic mindset, instead of accepting the inevitability of diabetes (and the use of multiple medications), we can think about avoiding the problem altogether. Fortunately, a simple way exists, and all it takes is carbohydrate restriction.

Summary: Dietary carb restriction was once acknowledged as the way to treat diabetes. It was forgotten with the rise of insulin and metformin. The current way prefers to cram all the excess glucose into cells, over the cells' objections (defensive insulin resistance). This does not alleviate the high rates of heart disease experienced by diabetics. But returning to the simple, dietary method offers a way to do it naturally.

Chapter 3: The HFLC Diet

The healthy man is the thin man. But you don't need to go hungry for it: Remove the flours, starches and sugars; that's all. ~ Samael Aun Weor

Is Glucose the Preferred Fuel?

As long as there is surplus glucose, insulin prevents the release of fat from adipocytes, by providing them with a constant supply of glycerol. This establishes a powerful pecking order. Glucose is burned first, and fats are only burned once glucose is depleted. Does this argue that glucose is the preferred fuel? If you asked Usain Bolt, or any other athlete who relies on explosive bursts of strength or speed in excess of what can be supported by the rate of oxygen-delivery, they would surely pick glucose over fat. Their muscles use stored glucose, and ferment large amounts of it to lactic acid in short bursts, to supplement their aerobic respiration. The result is a lot of energy produced rapidly, at the expense of efficiency. Following a short burst, they need to recover, clear the lactic acid, and establish new stores of glucose. Fats cannot be burned independent of oxygen, making them less ideal for quick bursts of speed.

By the age when type II diabetes is a relevant concern, intense athletic endeavors are well behind us. The type of sustained exercise best for our health is easily supported by a healthy respiratory system, and fats are an excellent fuel. When we embark on a hike of several hours duration, and are accustomed to burning fat, there is no need to eat anything while on the hike. Most us are carrying more than twenty pounds of fuel with us at all times, even if we are reasonably lean. But those whose metabolisms rely only on glucose may only have a few hundred grams of stored fuel, and will need to snack along the way, or make a quick adjustment to burning fat. Glucose, then, is not the most plentiful fuel, it is merely the first fuel used.

For another look at the question, let's review an obscure economic principle. Gresham's Law states that when two forms of money are forcibly given legal parity, the more valuable is driven out of circulation. It was first observed when gold or silver coins were debased, and people hoarded the good ones, while spending the debased ones, which continued to circulate. A modern example is when a small, poor country issues its own currency, and declares it to be on par with the US Dollar. They quietly flood the market with the local currency, but the people quickly learn which is more valuable, and hoard US Dollars, which fall out of circulation (except for private transactions). They freely spend the less valuable local currency, which is constantly in circulation. The lesson: The less valuable currency is spent first. The more valuable is stored for future use.

Returning to the question at hand, fat can be stored in large quantities, while glucose storage is limited to several hundred grams. Fat holds far more energy per weight than glucose, and glycogen is heavily hydrated, adding that much more weight. We even have cells whose primary function is to store fat, out of harm's way. Nothing like that exists for glycogen, which is stored in the liver and muscles. Once those stores are full, additional glucose is not stored. It is converted to fat, which can be stored much more efficiently. Further, glucose is slightly toxic. When in excess, the body needs to get rid of it. What better way to get rid of it than to burn it before burning fat? Likewise, alcohol and fructose are more toxic than glucose. They are therefore used as fuel for the liver before glucose. So the order of which fuel is used first is not indicative of the quality of that fuel, but rather its toxicity if left in circulation. In parallel with Gresham's Law, the more toxic fuel is used first, and the stable fuel is stored for future considerations, burned only after everything else is depleted.

Summary: More toxic fuels are burned first. Then, less toxic ones. Alcohol and fructose are burned first, then glucose, and fat last. Fat is only burned once the body is starved of carbs.

High Protein? No, High Fat

I once had a discussion with an old friend with diabetes, and he asked, "So is it just a high protein, low carb diet?"

"No," I answered him. "It's *high fat, low carb* (HFLC). Protein intake has to be moderate."

The discussion went in a different direction after that, and I suspect my twenty second pitch did not sway him. Like most everyone else, he had been conditioned to consider protein good, in any amount, and fat, bad.

A recent report in the news bore the headline, "Atkins diet can cause heart failure." Shocking, but once I read the first few lines, and saw it was pointing the finger at high protein consumption as the culprit, I shook my head and disregarded it. Atkins is not a high protein diet. Protein intake must be moderate, or the diet would be worthless, at best.

There is an important difference between protein and carbohydrates. Carbs are entirely non-essential in the diet. My health continues to improve, nearing three years since I cut my carbohydrate consumption to under twenty grams per day (versus the recommended 300 grams). If they were essential, surely I would suffer some kind of negative effect. Protein, on the other hand, is essential, up to a point. Estimates and circumstances vary, but something between fifty and a hundred grams of protein per day is necessary to replace amino acids that are broken down. Less than that, chronically, and the body begins to waste away. Much more than that, and excess protein is simply converted to glucose, or fat.

But protein must have the world's best public relations agent, because its image is uncritically good. In the minds of the people, protein is the dietary equivalent of the best off-road vehicle, the most agile snowboard, the lightest track shoes. It is what makes a man muscular, after all. We can debate whether we think actor Danny DeVito is made of carbs, or fat. But we probably imagine Arnold Schwarzenegger being made entirely of protein. When we think of the manliest food, we think steak. And not a small one. No self-respecting man wants to be seen eating a measly four ounce steak. The popular California burger chain In-N-Out Burger offers a rare option to take their burgers *Protein Style*. They even trademarked the name. Now, I don't want to seem ungrateful. I truly appreciate (and enjoy) the option of having my burger wrapped in lettuce instead of a bun. I'd even endorse the chain if they would cut the sugar out of their sauce. But I'm not happy about the name. It was probably developed with a focus group, who concluded that calling it high-fat low-carb would be problematic. This is only one example of the uphill battle to change people's perceptions and dial down protein consumption, while boosting fat consumption.

What's so bad about extra protein? Several things. In the amounts that have become glamorous (think of that 16 ounce

Porterhouse steak that is presented as a restaurant's signature entree), so much protein is consumed that the body cannot use but a small fraction of it. And what happens when the body is flooded with caloric nutrients it cannot use? It sends them to the liver, that poor, overworked organ. And the problem that follows should sound familiar. A pool of amino acids that should have been used over the course of a week is presented in one meal. The liver does its best, but such an overload has consequences. The liver converts most amino acids to glucose, until that too is in excess. The rest it converts to fat, and packages it into VLDL particles, which export it to adipocytes. The final outcome of eating that 16 ounce steak is no different than a small serving of protein, a plate of spaghetti, a frosted cake and a sweet dessert wine (although the steak will not produce the abrupt glucose spike).

I hope this clarifies that too much protein is not a good thing. And that the very concept high protein, low carb is self-contradictory. The high protein component is simply converted to carb. The diet I speak of is high-fat, low-carb. That scares a lot of people, probably including my friend mentioned in the beginning of this chapter. But this should not be so. The amount of fat stored as a result of this diet will be less than is stored by a high-carb, or high-protein diet, and it is normal to experience significant weight loss. A high-fat diet dispenses with intermediates, and directly provides the body the fuel it craves. It satisfies hunger in much lower amounts than other diets, resulting in less eating. It stimulates the central nervous system to expend energy, resulting in more doing. Less eating, more doing equals feeling good, losing weight, and being healthy.

To anyone unfamiliar with low-carb dieting, the first question might be, *How am I supposed to satisfy my hunger, if I can't eat a whole steak? No potatoes either? Because if you tell me it's tofu and salad, we're done. You can measure me for my coffin right now. That's preferable to tofu.* Bear with me. I would not have tolerated that, either.

The very word *fat* arouses a lot of anxiety today. I understand that perfectly well. Because for me, in a hurry to fix my diabetes before I had a chance to read extensively on the subject, it truly felt like diving into dark water without knowing whether there were rocks lurking just below the surface. There was only the word of the stranger sitting on the shore, and I couldn't be sure he was trustworthy. I made the dive, I surfaced, and am better for it, and would like to help make others' experiences easier. Mine is far from the first or only account of low-carb dieting, so we'll also review some noteworthy predecessors.

Summary: Excess protein is no different biochemically than spaghetti and a sweet dessert. Three ounces a day is about all you need. Fat is what satisfies hunger.

Ketosis and the Keto Flu

During periods of fasting, the body burns fat for fuel. And most organs and tissues are perfectly happy burning fat, but there are exceptions. Parts of the brain require either glucose, or lacking that, the ketone beta-hydroxybutyrate (BHB). When glucose is lacking, insulin goes quiet, and that signals the liver to turn fat into BHB. Even a smidgeon of insulin is enough to turn off ketone production, and what is in circulation disappears very quickly. It's interesting that even when the liver is insulin resistant in the sense that it won't take up glucose, it responds to the other effects of insulin, such as shutting off BHB production.

The presence of BHB is thus an excellent marker for the absence of circulating insulin. The state of fasting when BHB is being produced is referred to as *ketosis*. Those ancestors of ours who spent long winters subsisting on their fat reserves, supplemented by an occasional kill, were in ketosis for many months at a time.

A diet that deliberately eliminates carbohydrates and moderates protein intake, resulting in the production of BHB, is called a *ketogenic* diet. The person is adequately nourished, but is selectively starving the insulin response, and breaking the insulin resistance feedback loop. In addition to the health benefits of shutting down the feedback loop, a ketogenic diet is anti-inflammatory, and a hot research topic is the effect of ketosis on cancer prevention. Early signs are very promising.

There is widespread misunderstanding of ketosis in the medical community, probably because ketones are taught only in the context of diabetic ketoacidosis. Ketoacidosis is an out-of-control condition experienced only by insulin-dependent diabetics, where the total lack of insulin fails to check the liver's production of both glucose and BHB. The concentration of BHB can then top 20 mM, at which point it can acidify the blood. The condition is life-threatening, but is easily controlled with even a small amount of insulin. But the key lies in the numbers.

Table: Nutritional Ketosis is not at all like Ketoacidosis

	Blood BHB	Blood Glucose
Nutritional Ketosis	0.5 - 3.0 mM	Less than 150 mg/dl
Ketoacidosis	More than 20.0 mM	More than 240mg/dl

In the above table, nutritional ketosis occurs when BHB is in the range of 0.5 - 3.0 mM, with temporary spikes as high as 5.0 mM, after intense exercise. By contrast, ketoacidosis is characterized by BHB *ten times* as high as nutritional ketosis. Ketosis will not happen if blood glucose rises above 150 mg/dl (8.5 mM), whereas ketoacidosis occurs when the total lack of insulin results in excessive glucagon release, which raises glucose above 240 mg/dl (13 mM), more than twice normal. In other words, the margin of safety is actually a lot more for BHB than it is for glucose. Further, it is almost universally accepted that intermittent fasting can produce health benefits, so it's important to make the connection that periods of fasting *ARE* periods of controlled ketosis.

Most in the modern world have never had occasion to spend long periods of time burning fat instead of carbohydrates. So genes encoding the enzymes we need to burn fats, make ketones, etc., are idle. It would be wasteful to make those things, when they're never used. When a person suddenly goes into nutritional ketosis, everything has to be turned on, and that involves a period of adjustment. Other changes happen during the transition, related to the sudden drop in circulating insulin levels. Kidneys that had previously retained water now let it pass more freely. Some electrolytes are lost together with that water, and have to be replenished. The period of adjustment can be difficult for some people, and is sometimes called the *keto flu*. It's not really a flu, but at times, one may feel malaise comparable to a flu. Fortunately for me, the symptoms were relatively easy to manage, once I knew what to expect.

Every credible guidebook to ketogenic dieting for weight loss points out that the transition can be made slowly, to ease the difficulty. But for me, impatient as I was to rid my body of the excess glucose, a gradual approach was out of the question. From my perspective, allowing my microvasculature to continue to deteriorate for some time longer, simply so I could make an easy transition to nutritional ketosis, was a quaint concern. I was ready to endure some hardship. In retrospect, the hardest thing was not having a sense of normalcy, and not knowing what to expect. When trying to decide whether something was transitory, permanent, or something about my health going seriously awry, there was no standard against which to judge it. Even in my encounters with the medical system, there was no support. If I explained that I was pursuing nutritional ketosis, and the transition was proving difficult, the predictable answer would have been, "Then stop." The prescription pad, and food pyramid handout would surely have followed.

Shortly after I began to detect appreciable ketone levels in my urine (using urine dip sticks from the drug store), I felt weak and drowsy, for no apparent reason. Napping did not help, and soon I also found myself dizzy, irritable, and even slightly nauseous. I never actually threw up, but I came close on several occasions. When I sat down to eat, I was initially overcome by an unfamiliar, almost animalistic passion for the food. But after a few bites of fatty, low-carb food, I would abruptly hit a wall, and could not eat any more. In part, this was an adjustment I needed to make, because it now took far less food to satisfy my appetite. But there was something else at work during the transition. It was as if my body was craving carbs, and sitting down to eat made something inside me go crazy with that carb-passion. Then, after a few bites, that something realized it was not getting what it wanted, and went off to sulk. As weird as this felt, it was over in less than a week.

I quickly learned I could treat the lack of energy with a mineral supplement and a lot of water. I settled on a supplement with a physiologically appropriate mixture of sodium and potassium, supplemented by salts from the Great Salt Lake, called *Electrolyte*

Stamina Tablets, to deliver trace elements. The first time I took it, I was bed-ridden, and lacking the energy to sit up. Within fifteen minutes of taking it, I was on my feet. In a half hour, all my energy was back. I don't think I've ever experienced such a quick recovery from any malaise. All I needed to do was restore my fluids and minerals. This was another thing I could not explain to my doctor, who did not understand why I was experiencing my symptoms. She simply looked at my previous blood test, and seeing normal electrolyte levels, assumed nothing could have changed.

There were probably only a few days where the keto flu affected my disposition, and those were quickly remedied with the mineral supplement and water. Then, keto flu departed as suddenly as it came. I was quickly exercising again, with more energy than I ever had before. I no longer became drowsy in the afternoon (provided I had slept adequately, of course), and meals were again pleasant experiences.

Today, I will occasionally (once a month, or less) eat a meal with beans, or other nourishing food that puts me out of ketosis. I value nutritional variety as a way to ensure I am getting everything I need. Then, within a day or two, as I re-enter ketosis, I may experience an echo of the keto flu, which I treat with electrolytes and water as before.

Summary: Keto flu is the transition period, where the body adapts to using fat, which it probably has not done much in the past. Insulin levels drop, and fluid is lost, along with electrolytes. Water and mineral supplements overcome over this problem. But this is the time to be most cautious, as it's impossible to predict with certainty how your body will react. It might be mild, or it might be problematic. It also helps to have a doctor who supports what you're doing.

Eating High-Fat, Low-Carb (HFLC)

Think bacon and eggs, but without the toast. Avocado in an omelet is great, but hash-browns are out. Think heavy whipping cream in your coffee, but of course, no sugar, ever. Lots of butter in just about everything. Cooking with coconut oil, olive oil, avocado oil. Even bacon fat, when you have a lot left over. At first, I tried substituting steamed, mashed cauliflower for mashed potatoes, and it was awful. Watery, and insipid. But I soon learned I could make it acceptable by adding a lot of cheese. Or very good, with cheese, sour cream, and some garlic. Or downright delicious with all of the above, plus some crumbled bacon. I was making it highly satisfying by adding fat. If the fat disturbed me at all, it was offset by my certainty that diabetes was a far greater risk factor for heart attack and stroke than a little extra fat or cholesterol (the topic of the next chapter).

Another reservation might be that this kind of diet would make you feel bloated after a meal. Fortunately, that's far from the truth. Because cutting the carbohydrates, and only eating until full, eliminates all bloating and drowsiness after eating. Of course, eating a high fat diet makes me full a lot sooner, so I eat less overall. Once my insulin levels declined, and my leptin sensitivity came back, I felt transformed, as if by magic. I suddenly felt more energetic than I ever recall being, in my life. And it is trivial to keep my focus for many hours, where previously it could be a struggle.

There are easy tests that detect ketosis. At first, acetoacetate will appear in the urine, and can be detected with inexpensive dip sticks. But it is only an intermediate in the production of the relevant blood ketone, beta hydroxybutyrate (BHB). Eventually, as the body acclimates to the new diet, the acetoacetate will disappear, while BHB remains in the blood. After that transition, blood test strips very similar to those used for glucose measurements are needed for ketone quantification.

Mild ketosis is when BHB blood concentrations fall between 0.5 and 1.5 mM. For weight loss, 1.5 to 3.0 mM is considered optimal. I rarely exceed 2.0 mM, and usually only for a short time after intense exercise. Some who practice the ketogenic diet for weight loss consciously try to boost their ketones higher, to between 3.0 and 4.0 mM. They may burn more fat, faster, but the initial weight loss phase is already very quick. For me, it was forty pounds in about six weeks. Once an equilibrium weight is reached, weight loss ends as fast as it started, regardless. And a blood BHB level of 1.0 mM is already an indication that insulin is not active, which is the most important thing for a diabetic.

The breaking of diabetes happens as the insulin response goes idle. Ketosis is a good sign that this has happened, but it is not clear whether it is necessary. There are, however, other benefits attributed to the ketogenic diet, including far less incidence of irritable bowel syndrome, heartburn and GERD, Alzheimer's (often called type III diabetes), mental illness, depression, polycystic ovary syndrome, reduced cancer risk, and reduced heart disease risk. Ketosis has long been used to treat epilepsy, and before drugs for that purpose, was the standard treatment. The list is too long to evaluate each claim, and some of the benefits are no doubt associated with reduced glucose metabolism, and reduced insulin levels. Others may be attributable to the presence of BHB.

One popular term related to the HFLC diet is the *Paleo* Diet. It is based on the notion that before the rise of agriculture, and for most of our history, we did not have steady access to carbohydrates. It invokes the word *Paleolithic*, or "Old Stone Age," to describe a diet eaten by cavemen. The *Caveman Diet* is another popular term with a similar meaning. And there is considerable overlap between these and a ketogenic diet. The difference is that there is a strict definition of a ketogenic diet: It deprives the body of carbs, resulting in nutritional ketosis. However, there is no such strict definition of a Paleo diet. Every guru can create his own definition, based on his sense of what cavemen ate. For example, Paleo diets tend to accept honey as a sweetener, because cavemen had access to honey. But a ketogenic diet is not compatible with honey, or sugar in any presentation. Cavemen had access to ripe fruit on a seasonal basis. Does that mean the Paleo diet only allows fruit seasonally? Or does a particular interpretation allow fruit at any time? I doubt you'll find a consistent answer.

For healthy people, even a loosely defined Paleo diet will invariably be an improvement over the standard diet, and the differences might be considered quibbling. But for a diabetic, that's not the case. Just because something is natural, or organic, does not make it okay, if it further amplifies, or prolongs, the insulin resistance feedback loop.

Summary: A ketogenic diet results in burning fat. There will be traces of ketones in the blood, and this is a good thing. The terms Paleo and Caveman Diet are similar, and sometimes the same as a ketogenic diet. But they do not have strict definitions, and sometimes accept things not compatible with a ketogenic diet.

Carbohydrates and Human History

The singular event that triggered the rise of human civilization was the cultivation of grains, wherein carbohydrates became the staple food. Rice, wheat, barley, and rye were cultivated along rivers, and soon, history saw the rise of Egypt, Babylon, India and China. Even Central and South American civilizations were supported by the cultivation of grains. At the same time, human skeletons became smaller, and median lifespans decreased. Interestingly, the same source highlights that the median woman's pelvic inlet depth, which dictates the ease or difficulty of childbirth, decreased very dramatically at that time, and even today has not recovered its Paleolithic dimensions (Angel, (1984) *Paleopathology at the Origins of Agriculture.* Orlando: Academic Press, p. 51-73). So for women who wonder how their ancestors could have survived childbirth under primitive conditions, it was not always so difficult. It became difficult at the time of the Neolithic transition, when grains became the staple food. We see the same with modern Inuit women, who have an easy childbirth, if raised on the traditional diet. But if raised on a carbohydrate diet, the first generation develops exactly as all other modern women, and has a difficult childbirth.

In spite of these downsides, grain-fed civilizations prevailed in multiple places, over a short period of time. Why? The following thought experiment suggests that once it began, the transition to farming became unavoidable, and irreversible.

With the rise of farming, it quickly became necessary to invent a radical new concept: Land ownership. Tribes who hunted and killed a large animal probably felt ownership of that kill, but would not understand the concept of owning the live herd, or the land itself. But the farmer who spends long hours toiling in the field to produce a crop needs some assurance that come harvest time, the crop will belong to him. Mechanisms of governance developed to resolve land ownership disputes, and to protect groups of farms from marauding hunter-gatherers. Imagine what would happen when a group of hunter-gatherers came upon a field with a ripe, edible crop. They would help themselves to it, because they would not understand how anybody could own it. Or if the farmers were raising livestock, the hunter-gatherers might kill a cow, because it was what they always did. The probable response of the civilization is obvious to us: They would organize an army, and eliminate the threat to their livelihood. That is, they would kill the hunter-gatherers.

It's a given that intensive farming could support a far larger population than the hunter-gatherer lifestyle, and allow the organization of a sizeable army. And so over time, as civilization spread to all of the world's productive lands, the remaining hunter-gatherers either retreated to less hospitable environs, or were exterminated in clashes with farming societies. Eventually, most of the world's nomadic hunter-gatherers disappeared, as coexistence proved unworkable. This extended into the twentieth century. The only remaining holdouts live in marginal environments, where agriculture is not possible. In addition to the Inuit, the San people of the Kalahari Desert persist in an environment not suitable for agriculture. It is only natural, therefore, that the crops that allowed civilizations to arise and win conflicts with hunter-gatherers would continue to be the staples supporting those populations. To recap: One or several small groups of people may have first chosen to farm, and quickly had to invent civilization. Thereafter, everyone else either had to join the civilization, or die in clashes with it.

Some amount of meat nearly always entered the diet, with amounts varying according to the agricultural wealth of the society, but the staple food continued to be grain (or later, potatoes). It is unlikely that those societies faced anything like metabolic syndrome as a result of eating grains, given the poverty of the people, who faced constant hunger. In any event, given the hazards faced by those societies in the form of epidemics, contaminated water, and warfare, metabolic syndrome in middle age did not amount to an identifiable threat. We only see metabolic syndrome emerge in significant numbers after the age of fifty, and few people in those societies even lived that long.

It was only as societies became wealthier and more urbanized that obesity and its related problems began to appear. While the farmer's manual labor was enough to burn excess glucose, the urban professional lacked such exercise. The problem was exacerbated by the coincident development of refined flour. Now, blood glucose levels could rise quickly after a meal, spiking the insulin levels of the urban professional who had not managed to work off glycogen reserves left over from his last meal. One of the first societies to reach this level of wealth was Great Britain. As the problem of obesity spread, influential people began to look for relief from its associated health issues. One such man who became increasingly desperate to lose weight was William Banting.

Summary: The switch to farming worsened human health, but once underway, was irreversible. Farming gives rise to a structured society, that can exterminate outside threats like hunter-gatherers. Diseases of ageing only became relevant after societies became wealthy, and urbanized. Refined flour and sugar made their appearance in the same time frame.

William Banting and Robert Atkins

William Banting (1796-1878) struggled with his weight for many years. He consulted with many different doctors to try to find relief, to no avail. After failing with every other approach, he finally found a doctor named William Harvey, who prescribed an early version of the HFLC diet, and the results were staggering. Weight fell off him at an unprecedented rate, and his health was quickly restored. He felt so overwhelmed, and grateful, that he wrote a testimonial entitled the *Letter on Corpulence*. Reaction from the medical community was generally negative, and accusations were made that he had ruined his own health. However, he lived to the age of 82, which in the nineteenth century, speaks for itself.

Banting's diet became very popular, but over time, its public understanding became tainted by the medical system's insistence on deleting the high fat component, which Banting maintained was essential. Still, the Banting diet, in various forms, continued to be the standard method of weight loss until past the middle of the twentieth century. Banting faded from prominence, and his work was largely forgotten, save for epileptics, who found the HFLC diet effective at suppressing their seizures. Nobody thought to notice that epileptics of that time were not obese or diabetic.

As Banting's approach faded from memory, and obesity-related disease began its rise, a cardiologist who was himself struggling with his weight and health seized on the work of Dr. Alfred Pennington, who had *discovered* that a high fat low carb diet was indeed effective at combating obesity. He had only re-discovered Banting's diet (We could call it Harvey's diet, but Banting popularized it), but he had given it a patina of modern credibility. The name of the cardiologist was Robert Atkins, and so was born what we call the Atkins diet.

Atkins was the first to teach the ketogenic diet in its pure form, and used it with great success in his clinic. But in an echo of the reception Banting received, relations were never good between Atkins and the medical establishment. When he died after slipping on an icy sidewalk and hitting his head, stories were circulated to the effect that his diet was the cause. One wonders what it is that makes the medical system of multiple generations reflexively oppose dietary fat. Perhaps it is as simple as asking what a fat person has too much of. Obviously, it's fat. So telling him to eat more fat must sound as insane as a doctor telling me to keep eating carbs when I have diabetes. That much is understandable. Yet they continue to recommend carbs for diabetics, but discourage fat consumption for the obese, so the contradiction remains. And while a fat person may *store* too much fat, it is their insulin that directs their bodies to store too much fat. Invariably, they eat too much carbohydrate.

Atkins' publishers are alleged to have insisted he de-emphasize the high fat component of the diet, so those who find it through Atkins' books see it as a high protein diet, bringing us back to the PR problem in getting people to accept fat, and limit protein. Atkins recognized that excess protein was in effect slow-acting carb. Since Atkins re-popularized the ketogenic diet, the number of doctors who, having tried everything else and failed, swallowed their instinctive revulsion and found immediate success with Atkins, keeps growing. Researchers have taken up the science behind the ketogenic diet, and the body of work is evolving rapidly. Atkins preached the diet as a means of weight loss, and once achieved, taught his patients to find the right amount of carbohydrate for their own biochemistry. But since that time, it has emerged that there is no single measure associated with good health that is not enhanced by the ketogenic diet. BHB in the blood is anti-inflammatory, which is probably more cardio-protective than any medicine. Blood pressure declines as insulin-induced fluid retention and vascular smooth muscle hypertrophy goes away. HDL (controversially called *good cholesterol*) is known to increase.

With Atkins' message diluted in publication, it took another generation of authors, along with the emergence of the internet, blogs and videos, for the message to get out to a wide audience. Next, I'd like to single out several individuals who have emerged as leaders of the anti-carb movement, at least from my personal perspective.

Summary: The HFLC diet was first popularized by William Banting, in 1863. It was forgotten as the war on fat intensified, until Robert Atkins began to teach the same diet. Both were opposed by the medical establishment every step of the way, for their insistence on the importance of high fat.

Gary Taubes

Taubes has authored numerous books, the most pertinent of which was *Good Calories, Bad Calories*, a rigorously documented book exploring the history of today's health paradigms. In part one, he recounts the rise of the idea that fat caused heart disease, and the unscientific manner in which scientists, and then bureaucrats, accepted the theory in the face of contradictory evidence, and rejected any other, more plausible theory. In part two, he shows how the alternative view, that refined carbohydrates and sugar were responsible, was rejected out of hand, not because there was evidence to refute it, but because it was at odds with the accepted fat theory. If fat was declared guilty not only until proven innocent, but long afterwards, then sugar and refined carbs were declared innocent, long after being proven guilty.

In part three, Taubes traces the roots of our understanding of obesity, in the process debunking any notion that it is caused by an imbalance of calories in, versus calories out. Instead, the question we should ask is why the obese person eats more calories than he/she uses. The conventional model implies gluttony and sloth, but Taubes shows quite convincingly that it is not a moral failing, but a failing of the composition of the diet, or in some cases, genetics. Taubes debunks any notion that fat is inherently bad, and shows quite convincingly that it is carbohydrate intake that causes weight gain, precisely because of the involvement of insulin. One photograph shows a middle aged woman who had been an insulin-dependent type I diabetic for many years. Otherwise thin, she had two prominent, localized bulges of fat, one on each thigh, exactly where she had been injecting herself with insulin. There are numerous other examples, meticulously pulled from the historical record, that leave little room for doubt. As good as it is, some people felt the book was overly scientific, and insufficiently accessible to the general reader, so he produced a simpler version, called *Why We Get Fat: And What To Do About It*.

Robert Lustig

Lustig started his professional life as a pediatric endocrinologist, who saw progressively more obese children, suffering from many of the same maladies as older people. Eventually, he decided to delve into the biochemistry of obesity, and did a stint as a post-doctoral researcher in the field, before joining the faculty at the University of California, San Francisco. He combined his research with treating obese children, and played an important role in mapping the roles of insulin and leptin in regulating weight gain. He has a very popular video on Youtube, called *Sugar: The Bitter Truth* (if reading without the ability to hyperlink directly from the text, use code dBnniua6-oM), while his book, *Fat Chance*, documents the science and politics that has led to the present public health disaster. Not satisfied with that, he went on to study law, and is now involved in public policy initiatives, presumably to bring about changes in the guidelines.

Lustig's primary target is fructose. He once authored a paper that called fructose, "Alcohol without the buzz." In his many lectures, he maps out, in biochemical detail, how unlike glucose, fructose can only be processed by the liver, and is not converted to glucose or stored as glycogen. It reacts with proteins seven times as strongly as glucose, and creates one hundred times as many reactive oxygen species. A bolus of sugar, whether from a candy bar or a glass of fruit juice, floods the liver with far more fructose than it can utilize. Not only does this back up the uptake of glucose, it overwhelms the liver's mitochondria. The citric acid cycle becomes overwhelmed, and kicks out excess acetyl-CoA. Excess acetyl-CoA is converted to fat, which builds up and causes fatty liver disease, no different from alcoholic fatty liver disease. The newly synthesized fat spills out of the liver in the form of VLDL, still considered by some an important risk factor for heart disease (addressed in the next chapter).

Lustig goes so far as to call fructose a fat. Yes, he knows it's a carb, biochemically. He uses it as a device, to get across the point that fructose metabolism leads straight to fat. I must also credit Lustig for indirectly helping me resolve a puzzling issue I had with VLDL and triglyceride levels, even after my HDL had risen to what are considered protective levels. Until coming across his work, I had not fully appreciated the corollary of Lustig's assertion that fructose was as bad as alcohol: That alcohol is as bad as fructose.

Lustig does not put much stock into measurements of blood glucose, because in his words, "Once blood glucose changes, the horse is out of the barn." From his perspective, the patient is lost. And for a pediatrician, this is understandable. He wants to save the child's health, many years before diabetes develops. But from the perspective of a middle aged diabetic who did not want to be here, it can do no good to think this way. As I have learned for myself, we need not be lost, so long as we make appropriate changes to our eating habits.

I have adopted Lustig's recommendations for children. Sugar is banned outright at my house, even for the children. Beyond that, I have not imposed a strict ketogenic diet on my children, and allow carbs at a reduced level. But I am vigilant about not allowing frequent consumption of large amounts of carbs. I try to limit their circulating insulin levels, and the weight it causes them to put on.

Summary: "It's the fructose, stupid." At least from the perspective of increasing pediatric obesity, fatty liver, and diabetes. Lustig calls fructose, "Alcohol without the buzz," because the two are metabolized in exactly the same way.

Jimmy Moore and Eric Westman

Author and blogger Jimmy Moore is arguably today's most popular proponent of the HFLC diet. His story echoes so many others, and was driven by the need for weight loss from a high of 400 pounds. After experiencing futile cycles of trying to control his weight using guideline-based dieting techniques, he stumbled on the Atkins approach, and made a, *why not?* decision. The result was a loss of 180 pounds over one year, and a new life as the champion of the diet that gave him back his life. He has produced several books, frequently collaborating with Eric Westman, MD, Director of the Lifestyle Medical Clinic at Duke University Medical Center.

Moore and Westman deserve credit for popularizing the HFLC diet as much more than the weight loss technique championed by Atkins, even though Moore came across it for exactly that reason. And while Moore has a natural talent for bringing the message across to people, it is Westman who provides the medical background underpinning the diet. I own copies of *Keto Clarity* and *Cholesterol Clarity*, by Moore and Westman. Both are introductory books, written in an accessible style, and I regularly lend both to friends and acquaintances who have questions. Moore and Westman additionally run blogs, give lectures, and have an extensive presence on the internet, providing information about the HFLC diet.

Chapter 4: Just a Second, How About Heart Disease?

Public facts ... *must be picked, polished, shaped and packaged. Finally ready for display they the bear the marks of their shapers.* ~ Peter Conrad

The HFLC diet is such an obvious solution to diabetes that the only possible reason why every diabetic is not practicing it is because of what we've been taught about fat. And fat, heart disease, and cholesterol carry so much financial and political baggage that an unrestrained discussion would forcibly transform this into a book mostly on heart disease. And that would mostly duplicate what has been done very well by others (see **Appendix III**). I decided to maintain a tight focus on diabetes, and limited myself to one chapter on heart disease, with a separate discussion of the relationship between diabetes and heart disease. And in spite of that decision, I spent far longer on this section than any other, worried whether I had stated the case adequately. If I am not convincing, please consult the definitive works, for answers to your questions.

The Conflict Inherent in Scientific Practice

Distilled to its essence, the message of this section is that the prevailing wisdom about heart disease is entirely wrong. And it is understandable if this proves difficult to accept. "How could so many smart people be so wrong?" is the response I anticipate. So before I recount why science has it so wrong, I should probably make a case for how that is not only possible, but likely.

We've all been taught how science is supposed to work. A scientist formulates a hypothesis, and then designs experiments to test that hypothesis. But an experiment can never prove a hypothesis true. It can either prove the hypothesis false, or it can stand among other experiments that fail to disprove it, or disprove alternative hypotheses. The more attempts to disprove a hypothesis that fail, the stronger that hypothesis becomes, until at some arbitrary point in time, it is promoted to a *theory*. The rub lies in how sincere an attempt was made to truly disprove the hypothesis, and how honestly the data were collected, and interpreted.

The proponent of a theory has a duty to try his best to prove himself wrong. The only accountability imposed on a scientist is the expectation that if he fails to find an obvious flaw, a colleague will, and he will be discredited. If it were the effects of gravity on an unsupported object, the system would be foolproof, because contradictions would be glaring. But when gauging the probability of heart disease against something as complicated as myriad dietary factors, every hypothesis will confront apparently contradictory data points. While the obvious conclusion should be that no single factor is associated with every instance of heart disease, that would leave the field without a working hypothesis, and scientists without experiments to conduct. While there is value in cataloging facts, I've heard that contemptuously described as *butterfly collecting*. The prestigious work lies in developing an explanation that makes sense of those facts.

The Perils of the Ad-hoc Hypothesis

It is a capital mistake to theorize before one has data. Insensibly one begins to twist facts to suit theories, instead of theories to suit facts. ~ Sherlock Holmes (by Arthur Conan Doyle)

A theory is like a road map. Without it, one is lost amid conflicting and confusing data points that fail to form a tidy line or curve. But when informed by a road map, we can exclude from attention all roads not leading to our destination. In the same way, a theory is used to inform us which facts are probably true, and which ones can be dismissed as due to some error or other. And we fall precisely into the capital mistake described by Sherlock Holmes.

When data contradict a favored hypothesis, two outcomes are possible. One, the author admits the contradiction, and abandons the hypothesis, in the process taking a hit to his prestige. Alternatively, the scientist can dig in his heels, and continue to adhere to the original hypothesis, only adding a patch to it, to cover up the experimental failure.

Patches on hypotheses can be developed as needed, to explain away experimental failures, and are referred to as *ad-hoc* hypotheses. The *ad-hoc* hypothesis normally appears in the Discussion section of a scientific paper, where results are explained and integrated into the scientific mainstream. If an *ad-hoc* hypothesis happens to be right, it can lead to a new discovery. But how likely is this, given that it was conjured up without evidence, and was based only on one's faith in another theory that has just been proven wrong?

The tendency of science to cling to disproven hypotheses is universal. For instance, the cosmological Big Bang model does not work without invoking that 96% of the matter in the universe is a construct called dark matter. It has never been measured, and yet the allure of the model is such that it continues to inform our understanding of the universe. The danger is that if disproven hypotheses are not discarded, and proof of their being wrong is casually explained away without evidence, then there remains no viable way for that wrongness to be exposed, and corrected. This is the crux of the problem with the lipid and cholesterol hypothesis.

The Lipid Hypothesis

Like everyone of my generation, I was educated in the current framework of the lipid hypothesis. In fact, my principle reservation in adopting this diet was with boosting my fat intake. Bacon fat and lard? Fatty cuts of meat? Cream and butter? I was imagining drain pipes clogged with grease, the way they teach us (incorrectly) that cholesterol clogs arteries. This was the part where I felt like I was diving into dark water, hoping the assurance was true, that there were no rocks hiding below the surface. I no longer fear fat, or even saturated fat. As I'll discuss later, the magnitude of cardiovascular disease risk attributable to diabetes itself vastly exceeds any blood lipid.

There is a fatal logical flaw in the belief that a diet low in animal fat is heart healthy, and high levels of animal fat are unhealthy. Such diets get most of their calories from carbs, which are taken up by the liver, and converted to fat. And here's the dirty little secret: *The liver does not make olive oil.* It makes animal fat, with a similar composition as other forms of animal fat, about 40% of which is saturated. The only difference when eating carbs is that the liver has to work harder to make the fat, resulting in stress and fat buildup in the liver.

Since the body makes its own saturated fat from carbs, is there something special about *dietary* saturated fat, that leads to higher cholesterol? The liver is the principal factory that makes cholesterol, and dietary fat bypasses the liver entirely. It goes straight from the gut to muscles and/or adipocytes, so it is not the liver's principal fuel source. An objection at this point might be that fat can later leave adipocytes, and return to the liver. Indeed it can, and it does. The vesicles that carry it back to the liver are known as HDL, the number of which increases on a high fat low carb diet, precisely so adipocytes *can* send fuel to the liver. HDL is often called *good cholesterol*, and while that *ad-hoc* hypothesis has no independent supporting proof, no evidence even begins to suggest that HDL causes heart disease.

Lastly, is saturated fat some sort of special starting material, used by the liver to make cholesterol? Absolutely not, even apart from the fact that the liver makes plenty of saturated fat, if fed carbs. The liver makes cholesterol using a long pathway, and the starting material is none other than the universal metabolic intermediate, acetyl-CoA. Every fuel that is burned for energy by mitochondria becomes acetyl-CoA before it enters the citric acid cycle, and is available for cholesterol production. So technically, this includes dietary sources of saturated fat, but it also includes every other fuel. So where does this anti-fat notion come from? Here follows a condensed history:

The medical community gave William Banting a very hostile reception when he published his *Letter on Corupulence*, so it goes back at least as far as the mid-nineteenth century. If one is inclined to give them the benefit of the doubt, it is useful to point out that this same medical community vigorously rejected Ignaz Semmelweis' simple demonstration that disinfecting the hands could save the lives of new mothers infected by their obstetricians. Even when Robert Koch proved that germs caused cholera and tuberculosis, the medical community was very slow to come around. So the hostility of the reception does not imply wrongness of the idea, only its non-conformity to existing beliefs.

The underlying bias against animal fat was exploited, and probably cemented, by the marketing campaign supporting the launch of partially hydrogenated vegetable oils. Hydrogenation of vegetable oils was first undertaken to make them suitable for the manufacture of soap. In the process, it was found that partial hydrogenation could make a softer product, roughly comparable to lard. That product was launched in 1911, under the name *Crisco*.

Cookbooks using Crisco in all their recipes were given away free when buying Crisco shortening, and extensive advertising touted the health advantages of vegetable-derived shortening over animal fats. How true was the claim? Today, we refer to partially hydrogenated vegetable oils as *trans fats*. If there is one fat that is indisputably bad for heart disease, it is trans fat. But the message of the campaign stuck, establishing in the public mind the idea that vegetable oils were healthier than animal fats. And since saturated fatty acids account for up to 40% of animal fat but are scarce in vegetable oils, it was assumed that saturated fat was the unhealthy component. In other words, it was an inference, based on a bias.

In principle, a scientific hypothesis derived from an advertising campaign is no better or worse than any other, but it carries more clout if accompanied by a mechanistic explanation. And an American scientist named Ancel Keys, also the inventor of the army's K-ration, married saturated fat with cholesterol, which had already garnered interest. Post-mortem examinations as far back as the nineteenth century often showed arteriosclerotic plaques that narrowed the blood vessels in the heart at specific locations. Dissection of those plaques turned up cellular debris, the remnants of old clots, and cholesterol (later found to be oxidized). This led to the hypothesis that cholesterol caused the disease. The hypothesis soon hit a snag, when it was found that dietary cholesterol had no impact on blood cholesterol. Keys stepped in, and argued that animal fat leads to elevated cholesterol, which leads to heart disease. The only thing missing was proof that animal fat leads to elevated cholesterol, or heart disease.

To create his proof, Keys launched a study later known as the Seven Countries study, the first version of which was published in 1953 (J. Mount Sinai Hospital 1953, 20:118-139). Keys tallied the saturated fat in all food sold (called disappearance data) in 22 countries, versus reported heart attack death rates. He then selected six countries, later expanded to seven, and excluded all others. He never explained why he picked those seven countries, but as it happens, his choice produced the best possible fit with the dietary fat and heart disease hypothesis. The earliest critics of his work objected to his selective use of available data (Yerushalmy and Hilleboe, American Epidemiological Society, April 5, 1957). Selecting only seven countries smacked of cherry-picking data to support a preconceived notion. One could have chosen a different set of seven countries, including France and Switzerland (where data were as good as any), and claimed the exact opposite: That saturated fat was protective against heart disease. The honest approach would have been to analyze all twenty two, but that produced no discernible trend.

Even if Keys had stuck to all twenty two countries, the study would not have been valid, as it suffered from too many methodological problems. First and most lethal, was that Keys only looked at saturated fat consumption, and ignored sugar. The seven countries he ended up choosing had identical trends in sugar and fat consumption, meaning either one could be relevant (or both; or neither). A legitimate study would have applied the same statistical analysis to sugar as it did to fat (multivariate regression). Keys never explained why he ignored sugar, and as his detractors point out, he was a vocal proponent of the fat hypothesis before the study even began. That his conclusion matched his preconception is hardly shocking, since he systematically excluded any data that could have undermined it. Additional problems included very wide international variability in the standards of reporting deaths, whether from heart attack or other causes. For instance, overall deaths were actually lower in those countries in the study that reported higher heart disease death rates. Any effect Keys reported could be due entirely to differing standards for reporting the causes of death.

Rationing during World War II led to the development of inexpensive margarine, which is of course partially hydrogenated vegetable oil, or trans fat. The advent of television commercials in the post-war years led to widespread acceptance of margarine, and by the time Keys' studies began, it was a significant dietary factor. Keys never made an effort to control for trans fat consumption, despite being warned to do so. The argument against trans fat dates back at least that far, with Professor Fred Kummerow leading the way, objecting that cells would not recognize those artificial molecules, and would not be able to process them correctly. Today, we know this to be true, as mitochondria cannot metabolize trans fats, and become gummed up by their remnants. If mitochondria in the heart are disabled by the remnants of trans fats, the heart is forced to produce energy by accelerated glycolysis, which leads to excessive lactic acid accumulation, and necrosis of heart tissue.

Kummerow also established that it was oxidized cholesterol that was present in the plaques associated with heart disease, and we'll return to that point later.

Criticism of Keys' work was widespread. In other circumstances, and all things being equal, the study would have been quickly forgotten. But all things were not equal. Keys soon won over the establishment, and in 1961, found himself on the cover of Time Magazine, with his hypothesis hailed as a breakthrough answer to heart disease. This gave him an almost legendary status in his field, and enabled him to intimidate dissenters into silence.

Keys' dominance was challenged in 1972, when King's College Professor John Yudkin published *Pure, White and Deadly: The Problem of Sugar.* In it, he linked increasing sugar consumption to the increasing rates of heart disease, obesity, diabetes, and of course, dental cavities. Yudkin was widely criticized for the same fundamental error made by Ancel Keys, namely not controlling for other factors. Ironically, the loudest voice condemning Yudkin was none other than Ancel Keys. Keys apparently saw no irony in condemning Yudkin for the same error that plagued his own work, nor explained why the same error should invalidate Yudkin's work, but not his own. What followed was a public war of words between Yudkin and Keys, whose fat and cholesterol hypothesis was suddenly at risk of being pushed off center stage. If Keys ever had any intention of analyzing his data for the role of sugar, it now became impossible from a practical perspective. For him to retract in such a public battle would have meant career suicide. And as detailed in the documentary movie, **Sugar Coated**, the sugar industry understood the threat posed by Yudkin's work, and fought back with an extensive public relations campaign. They also extended financial and political backing to natural allies, including Ancel Keys and Fred Stare, founder of the Department of Nutrition at the Harvard School of Public Health. Stare was a frequent guest on news shows, where he denied sugar posed any dangers, and that the only public health problem in America is that, "People eat too damn much."

At roughly the same time, heart bypass operations became more common, and heart surgeons observed first hand the yellow plaques in the arteries of those with heart disease. This seemed to confirm the observations of post-mortem reports, boosting the link between cholesterol and heart disease. Fred Kummerow's observation that it was actually oxidized cholesterol was set aside and ignored, because nobody understood its significance. And the presence of multi-layered old clots in those same plaques was also ignored, because it did not lead to any obvious conclusions.

Politics soon entered the fray, with the McGovern commission hearing all sides, listening only to Keys' side, and launching the anti-fat campaign still in effect today. The reduction in fat intake recommended by the McGovern commission was implemented exactly as mandated, but heart disease rates exploded. But the results seemed not to matter. Once the fat narrative was in place, competing ideas such as Yudkin's sugar hypothesis were selectively ignored, or attacked. The last thing anybody seemed to want was a return to the chaos of the time when the experts had to admit to being ignorant. Least of all, the experts themselves.

What finally put me at ease with respect to eating fat was putting risk factors into perspective. Multivariate regression analysis can isolate individual factors, and identify the relative risks they pose. After smoking and high blood fibrinogen levels (propensity to form clots), diabetes is the single biggest risk factor for heart disease (BMJ 1997, 315:722). No other risk factor even comes close. Single blood lipid factors do not even rank as statistically significant. The top priority for every diabetic must be breaking the feedback loop of increasing insulin resistance, and increasing insulin levels. This poses by far the greatest danger to our health, and is not improved at all by diabetes drugs and/or insulin, which transfer glucose toxicity from the blood to cells. So let's consider the possibility that it could be the act of over-stuffing our livers with carbs that is the problem.

Summary: There was always a bias against animal fat, which contains higher amounts of saturated fat than other fats. Ancel Keys decided animal fat causes elevated cholesterol, and selected data to support a link to heart disease. For his efforts, his face was on the cover of Time magazine, and his ideas were widely embraced. After that, the question was treated as settled.

But Cholesterol!

About twenty percent of the body's cholesterol is estimated to come from the diet, and eighty percent is made by the liver. The liver will adjust how much it makes, based on how much one consumes, to ensure there is enough for the body's needs. The net effect of the liver compensating how much it makes is that dietary cholesterol seems to have no impact on blood cholesterol. The only way to naturally prevent the liver from making any cholesterol is to stop eating altogether. Permanently. Some time after you die of starvation, your liver will indeed stop making cholesterol. This point bears repeating: Short of starvation, or liver failure, there is no *natural* way to make the liver stop synthesizing cholesterol. Eat more cholesterol, and the liver will reduce the amount it makes by a corresponding amount. Eat less, and the liver will make more.

We're instinctively afraid of cholesterol, even though it's a natural component of our bodies, so here's a question: If a person over age fifty experiences a natural drop in their cholesterol, can that person expect to live longer? You probably guessed that was a leading question. The answer is an emphatic *no*. Quite the opposite. A drop in cholesterol is a very strong predictor of early death (from the Framingham study). The reply is that the liver of the afflicted person was obviously somehow diseased. In other words, the person was sick in some other way. And as we'll see later, that is probably indeed the case. A sick liver makes for a sick person, and causes elevated heart disease risk. Especially when that liver is sick from a chronic carb overload.

But why does the liver keep making so much cholesterol, until it is literally too sick to do so? If cholesterol is so bad, why is a healthy liver so determined to keep the body so well stocked with it? Every important process is tightly regulated, and cholesterol is no different. Cholesterol is an essential component of the body. Without it, your cell membranes would all rupture, and you'd be dead in a second, flat. The body needs quite a lot of cholesterol to function properly. The brain is the first to suffer if cholesterol is lacking, and many of those who take statin drugs experience cognitive defects. Steroid hormones are made from cholesterol. Cholesterol is needed where wounds are healing. You are composed of cells, and cells are defined by membranes, which contain a lot of cholesterol. Those with naturally low cholesterol levels are prone to cancer, heart disease, and stroke. When patients are hospitalized with heart attack symptoms, and their cholesterol is measured at the hospital, it comes out lower than the average for the population as a whole. If you have doubts, don't take my word on it. Read the books I've listed in Appendix III.

In the cartoon version of the cholesterol story that many doctors continue to recount to their patients when ordering blood tests, cholesterol clogs arteries like grease clogs up drain pipes. Those cartoons are evocative because we can all imagine clogged drains, but that popular version is entirely wrong: The grease-in-a-drain analogy is impossible. Arterial plaques are sealed off from the blood by a contiguous layer of endothelial cells. In other words, the plaques, which contain a lot of cellular debris, old clots layered one on top of another, and oxidized cholesterol, are *under the skin*, so to speak. They also occur at very localized spots, never stretching beyond the rough length of a healing wound on the artery wall. Even the largest plaques, that form a ring around the entire inner diameter of the artery, are very short along its length. Grease in a drain forms deposits along the entire inner surface of the pipe, and over long stretches. Something entirely different is at work in arteries.

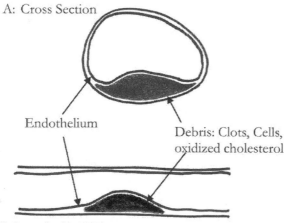

A: Cross Section

Endothelium

Debris: Clots, Cells, oxidized cholesterol

B: Longitudinal View

What follows is a summary of the current thinking in the field of cholesterol, although even the current thinking does not reflect the evidence. It continues to be based on the belief that blood cholesterol somehow causes arterial plaques, and ad-hoc hypotheses are added to patch over the holes in the idea.

Fats and cholesterol do not travel through the blood in isolation. Blood is water based, while fats are oily, and would form droplets if they circulated freely. Instead, they are packaged up into particles containing fat, cholesterol, and about 100 protein molecules per particle. The particles are known as *lipoproteins*, from *lipid*, meaning *fat*, and proteins. The particles are oily on the inside, but water soluble on the outside. Blood is sorted in a centrifuge, and particles are separated by how much they sink or float (determined by their density). LDL stands for low density lipoprotein, while HDL stands for high density lipoprotein. In addition, there are very low density lipoproteins (VLDL), and chylomicrons, sometimes called ultra low density lipoproteins. These designations are arbitrary, and carry over from their original identification using the centrifuge. As we'll see later, LDL encompasses many different particles, whose characteristics are as different as night and day. Lipoproteins also exist with intermediate densities, which do not match the classical lab profiles, so we know little about their properties. I will introduce the various particles and their roles, before addressing their status as *ad-hoc* hypotheses.

HDL is said to be good for you, and LDL is said to be bad. The latest hypothesis is that the smallest, densest forms of LDL are the truly bad ones, while large, fluffy, cuddly LDL particles might lick your face, but would never bite you. But if the bad ones are dense, doesn't that make them more like the *good* HDL? Chylomicrons are considered harmless, but have ultra-low density, closer to VLDL, which is considered bad. In short, there appears to be no simple rule relating particle density to whether that particle wears a white or black cowboy hat.

If there is a rule for hat color, it would be that particles destined for the liver are good, while those leaving the liver full of triglycerides are potentially bad, depending on how long they circulate. But note that if a lot of particles are leaving the liver, that is confirmation that the liver is working overtime to produce them. And if they are destined for the liver, then that liver is not under stress having to make fat.

VLDL: VLDL is produced by the liver, and is loaded with liver-produced triglycerides, and also some cholesterol. It is a big particle with an oily core, surrounded by a membrane. A single copy of the Apo B protein is on each VLDL particle, together with about 100 other proteins. VLDL travels through the body, and delivers its fat where needed. How does the VLDL particle know when to release fat? It doesn't. The particle is not alive, like cells are. It's simply a ball of oil, packaged up in a way that allows it to flow through blood. It's the cells who know when they're hungry, and make the enzyme *lipase*, which travels to the nearest small blood vessel, parking itself on the inner surface. That enzyme works within the lipoprotein, to break fatty acids apart from glycerol, so the free fatty acids can easily cross cell membranes.

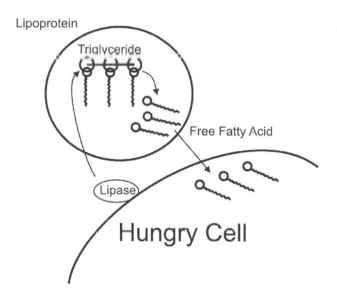

If there is no demand for fat, there is no lipase, and the VLDL particle happily continues its journey. As its fat reservoir is consumed, the VLDL particle shrinks and becomes denser, and cholesterol makes up a greater percentage of its cargo. It can deliver that cholesterol where needed, for instance at sites of wound healing. As it shrinks, at some arbitrary point it officially becomes an LDL particle.

LDL: LDL is thought to be VLDL that has lost some of its cargo, and continues to circulate. The considerable variation in the types of particles that constitute LDL has lead to their classification as either pattern A or pattern B LDL.

Pattern A LDL: The description of pattern A LDL sounds to me a lot like VLDL. They are large particles, and have a low density. It might be considered a simple continuation of VLDL, after it has lost some fat, or the contents may be present in different proportions. However, pattern A LDL is considered harmless, whereas VLDL is considered a risk factor.

Pattern B LDL: For reasons unclear to me, VLDL is said to mature into pattern B LDL, but not pattern A LDL. Possibly it is only a matter of numbers, and if VLDL levels are high, the number of particles will be high, leading to an eventual elevation in pattern B LDL. Pattern B LDL particles are small, hard, dense, and sticky. They are depleted of most of their fat, so the cargo is enriched for cholesterol. They have a long life in circulation, and that plus their small size makes their cholesterol very prone to oxidation. To me, pattern B LDL seems like a forgotten particle that should have been mopped up somewhere along the line, but it may have lost its surface markers, and the system lost track of it.

When drug reps present doctors with illustrated diagrams intended to explain the causes of heart disease, it is not the grease-in-a-drain picture they portray. They show an LDL particle (they don't specify pattern B LDL) traveling through the blood, then for no apparent reason, suddenly making a ninety degree turn, invading a blood vessel wall, burrowing its way past the endothelium and into the space beneath, and initiating the formation of a plaque. How multiple, layered clots also get into the plaque is never addressed. Also, recall that lipoproteins are inanimate balls of grease, without any capacity to control their own movements. For the hypothesis to work, the particle would have to move like an amoeba, and project pseudopods into the lumen, which it could then use to pull the rest of itself inside. That picture is inconsistent with an inanimate and inflexible pattern B LDL particle.

I will shortly review a plausible model for the development of heart disease that involves repeated injuries to the arterial endothelium. If pattern B LDL plays any role, it could be by sticking at sites of injury that are quickly covered up by new endothelial cells. With a core of oxidized cholesterol, it could be resistant to the natural processes that would otherwise clean it up.

Pattern B LDL levels correlate well with elevated triglycerides. Glucose, fructose, or alcohol are taken up by the liver and converted to triglycerides, and transported by VLDL, which matures to pattern B LDL, and as the model goes, contributes to plaque formation. The problem in evaluating pattern B LDL is the lack of data on a population-wide scale. Techniques exist that count the number of LDL particles in a blood sample (from which an inference can be made about their size), but it is rare to find a doctor who would order the test.

Chylomicrons: These particles assemble at the interface between gut cells and circulation. Fat and cholesterol consumed in the diet are packaged up, and the particles bypass the liver entirely. They deliver their contents to peripheral tissues, especially muscle and fat. Chylomicrons are short-lived, and blood tests are done while fasting, so chylomicrons do not factor into blood cholesterol measurements. This implies that dietary fat has no impact on blood cholesterol. Indeed, the data are challenging to proponents of the fat hypothesis, who often respond that high levels of chylomicrons deliver enough fat to satisfy cells' appetites, so those cells are not as hungry for carb-derived triglycerides from the liver in the form of LDL. This is said to lead to elevated circulating LDL. In practice, LDL elevations in response to the HFLC diet are slight or none. And the HFLC diet strongly skews LDL to the harmless pattern A variety.

HDL: HDL particles have different surface markers than the VLDL series. HDL particles collect fats and cholesterol from peripheral tissues, most significantly fat cells, and return them to the liver. So when there is a strong net flow of fat from adipocytes to the liver, as there is on the HFLC diet, HDL will be elevated, as it has to be.

HDL delivers fat and cholesterol to the liver, and thereby takes them out of circulation. In addition, HDL *bumps* into other lipoproteins in the course of its travels, and regularly donates some of its surface proteins to those particles, like a car that scrapes against yours *donates* some of its paint. If the bad pattern B LDL particles are lost, forgotten particles that continue to circulate indefinitely, then the result of a collision with HDL would be the pattern B LDL particle picking up an HDL marker, eventually leading to its uptake by the liver, and clearance from the system. The cholesterol hypothesis often takes things further, arguing that since HDL acts as a scavenger, it can collect fats and cholesterol from anywhere in the body, even from under the endothelium of artery walls. Some versions even suggest that HDL can wave a wand, speak an incantation, and dissolve atherosclerotic plaques residing under that arterial skin. Magical properties such as these should be viewed with a healthy dose of skepticism.

High HDL is considered protective against heart disease, but there is no direct evidence in its favor, just as there is no direct evidence against VLDL and pattern B LDL. The case for HDL rests entirely on the following *ad-hoc* hypothesis:

> *We know that saturated fat and cholesterol cause heart disease, and since the French eat very high amounts of saturated fat and have high cholesterol but have the lowest heart disease rates in Europe, another factor must be at work, protecting them. The French also have very high HDL, so that's what it must be.*

The case for HDL being protective is only valid if saturated fat and cholesterol are truly the causes of heart disease. The French have high HDL and low heart disease, so we at least know that HDL is not a cause of heart disease, but this does not prove HDL is protective. Malcolm Kendrick, whose work I'll cover shortly, points out that when analyzed by multivariate regression, HDL does not rise above noise as an independent predictive factor for heart disease. So the *ad-hoc* hypothesis fails, just as the parent hypothesis failed.

Lipoprotein	Character Description	Source
HDL	Superhero	Fat from adipocytes to liver
VLDL (Triglyceride)	Assistant Villain	Carbohydrates
LDL pattern A (large, light)	Wrongly Accused	Mix of sources
LDL pattern B (small, dense)	Arch-Villain	Old VLDL particles (carb)
Chylomicrons (ULDL)	Innocent Bystander	Dietary fat

The Fat Cycle:

One of the hallmarks of metabolic syndrome and diabetes is a low HDL/triglyceride ratio (VLDL and triglyceride are often used interchangeably). In other words, HDL is low, triglycerides are high. This has led some to use that ratio as an important health marker, when it is really only a dietary marker.

A liver accumulating fat from too much carb in the diet is not importing fat from adipocytes (which are not releasing fat). Accordingly, the vesicle that transports fat from adipocyte to liver (HDL) will be low. That liver is constantly exporting as much fat as it is able, in the form of VLDL particles, loaded with triglycerides, which will be high.

By contrast, when the liver is starved of dietary carbohydrates, it is not exporting any fat, and instead has to import fat from adipocytes. Therefore, that person will have very low VLDL, and very high HDL. But before we conclude that the lipid factors are themselves the health determinants, let's remember that the same person will have very low insulin levels, low liver inflammation, and nearly no fat in the liver. Suddenly, we have two explanations that both fit within the same framework, and to separate those, scientists employ a statistical technique called multivariate regression (next).

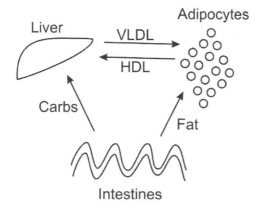

Figure: The Fat Cycle. Above the amounts needed for energy, fat from the intestines travels to adipocytes, whereas carbs travel to the liver. There, carbs are converted to fat and transported to adipocytes in VLDL. If carbs are in short supply, fat is transported from adipocytes to the liver in HDL. The ratio of VLDL to HDL may merely be an indicator of which way fat is traveling. Indirectly, it also speaks to the health of the liver.

Critiquing the Cholesterol Hypothesis:

A valid hypothesis, it is said, starts obscure, and changes little as it withstands test after test, until it is eventually accepted. The cholesterol hypothesis, by contrast, started off with maximum fanfare, and then proceeded to fail every test designed to validate it. But instead of being discarded, it was always re-formulated with a new set of assumptions, tailored to explain the latest failure. The only continuity between today's cholesterol hypothesis and the original is the unwavering belief that cholesterol must play a major role in the development of heart disease. Today's latest thinking on pattern B LDL is embraced by many advocates of the HFLC diet, as the theory validates the diet, which drastically reduces pattern B LDL. But that does not constitute evidence in support of the theory.

Now it's time to turn to the work of one of the most prolific critics of the cholesterol hypothesis, Dr. Malcolm Kendrick. Kendrick started out as a general practitioner who was slowly drawn into the field, and eventually became a *de-facto* specialist on the epidemiology of heart disease. First, a one-minute video that summarizes the case very succinctly: *Cholesterol and Heart Disease* (Youtube code i8SSCNaaDcE). Kendrick presents data taken from the World Health Organization's very large MONICA study, done on 32 countries from across Europe. Kendrick also includes the Australian Aborigines, who have the lowest cholesterol of any people, but are afflicted with the highest risk of heart disease. The Swiss, with the highest cholesterol in the MONICA study, have close to the lowest rate of heart disease. In between, there is no correlation between the two, and if anything, the data may imply a weak *inverse* correlation. Very low cholesterol results in very high heart disease risk, and very high cholesterol results in reduced heart disease risk. Kendrick will not commit to the inverse relationship, as the data are weak. As an afterthought, the people with the highest cholesterol ever measured for a population are the Masai of Africa, who have essentially no heart disease.

In a more detailed video, Kendrick details ten contradictions, each of which on its own should disprove the cholesterol hypothesis (Youtube code 8ls9HWRxvMo). Each of the ten is worthy of comment, but to keep things moving along, I'll confine myself to two.

The first contradiction looks at the actual risk factors for or against heart disease, ranked by their predictive power (BMJ 1997, 315:722). At the top of the list is previous heart attack, which only means the person's heart is already sick. Roughly tied for second are smoking and elevated fibrinogen, the clotting factor. The fibrinogen result tempts one to the conclusion that propensity to form clots is the cause of heart attacks, but other possibilities also have to be considered, since fibrinogen rises together with many other risk factors. And smoking seems bad for just about every morbidity.

Diabetes is close behind smoking and fibrinogen, but blood glucose does not even rank as significant. How so, since diabetes is diagnosed by high blood glucose. Kendrick does not comment, but I will: A diabetic without hyperglycemia is either following a HFLC diet (too few of us to show up in the numbers, and are we even diabetics anymore?), or is using a combination of diabetes drugs to move glucose out of their blood and into their cells. Mostly liver cells. The diagnosis of diabetes continues to be associated with heart disease risk, yet the control of blood glucose does not alleviate it. This provides further support for the notion that treating diabetes with drugs either does not reduce the risk, or the treatment contributes to the risk.

At the bottom of the list, with little to no statistical significance, are all the traditional risk factors. None of LDL, triglycerides, and even HDL, have any predictive power. Pattern B LDL was not included, as there is a lack of data, but high triglycerides are said to predict pattern B LDL. The only limitation of a study such as this that comes to mind is that combinations of putative risk factors could yet produce significant results, where individual factors do not.

The second contradiction cited by Kendrick is a comparison of heart disease rates and risk factors between Japan and Russia. Blood pressure, cholesterol, and smoking rates are all within a few percent of each other. And yet the Russians have 1,800% more heart disease (Ueshima, H. 2007. J. Atherosclerosis and Thrombosis 14:278-286). To be sure, there are many societal and even genetic differences between Russians and Japanese, so it is not trivial to isolate one causal factor. But whatever the explanation, it is not cholesterol, smoking, or high blood pressure. Vodka consumption comes to mind, and excessive alcohol consumption is famous for stressing the liver. But the magnitude of the difference calls for additional factors. Kendrick favors chronic stress, caused by a history of societal disruptions, and cites examples in other cases, to establish a correlation. We'll return to that topic later.

Kendrick's book on the subject is called *The Great Cholesterol Con*. Other significant works that debunk the cholesterol hypothesis include:

Good Calories, Bad Calories, by Gary Taubes

The Cholesterol Myths, by Dr. Uffe Ravnskov

Fat Chance, by Dr. Robert Lustig

For those wanting a lighter introduction to the subject, the irreverent documentary movie *Fat Head* by Tom Naughton presents a comical look at the question, with a lot of quality information.

Even with all of the above information, I concede that a normal reaction will be to shrug with skepticism. I too was drilled with the cholesterol hypothesis for so many years that it was a formidable obstacle. For those who want to read the whole sordid history of how the erroneous hypothesis developed, it is chronicled in extraordinary detail in the definitive book on the subject: Gary Taubes' *Good Calories, Bad Calories*. Your view of scientists as dispassionate and objective will not emerge intact.

The final objection I had, and therefore anticipate from my audience, pertains to all those widely publicized clinical trials of cholesterol-lowering statin drugs we hear about. If lowering cholesterol can lower heart disease risk, doesn't that kind of prove that cholesterol plays a role in heart disease? That discussion follows, with the concession that it would indeed prove it, if it were true.

Summary: The body needs a lot of cholesterol to function properly, and the liver makes what it needs. The cholesterol in arterial plaques is oxidized, and not the same as the cholesterol as the body needs. Further, plaques are underneath the equivalent of skin on the insides of arteries. That rules out a model of clogging arteries like grease in a drain. Saturated fat elevates good cholesterol (HDL), while only a subset of LDL is considered truly bad. That is, very old, small, hard, oxidized, sticky particles called pattern B LDL, associated with high carbohydrate consumption. A very large body of literature is reviewed, that debunks the cholesterol hypothesis, and the saturated fat supposition that seems to go along with it.

Statin Drugs

150 people die every year from being hit by falling coconuts. Not to worry, drug makers are developing a vaccine. ~ Jim Carrey

Scientific opinion on statins is a lot more divided than most people realize. Select individual trials have reported improvement in the rates of death by heart attack, although not in overall death rates. And accusations abound that only positive trials were ever reported, while the majority were simply buried, in effect cherry picking those trials that return positive results by chance alone. I can't judge those accusations, either way. When a trial is underwritten by a pharmaceutical company, the data belong to them, and they have the prerogative to publish or not publish. They can cite any number of reasons why a given trial is not valid, and outsiders have no standing to force the issue. All the same, the single independently funded study on statins (ALLHAT-LL) found no benefit of any kind.

Another complaint is the reporting of relative benefit, rather than absolute benefit. That means if one arm of a trial reports one heart attack in 100 patients, while the other arm reports two in 100, the absolute benefit is 1%, but the relative benefit is 50%, which gets the headline. But it's only a 50% benefit if you're among the two who get the heart attack, not if you're among the 98 who did not, and received no benefit. It would require identifying those two in advance, and only giving the drug to them, while sparing the other 98, in order to honestly call it a 50% benefit. It's presently impossible to make such accurate predictions, and would also drastically reduce the market for the drug. But every statin study has reported relative benefit. Lastly, statin trials never report overall mortality rates, and critics say that no statin trial has ever produced an overall mortality benefit. So even if a trial reports a benefit in death by heart attack, subject to the qualifications above, that benefit is offset by other causes of death.

To further complicate matters, even in the one group where most agree statins provide some benefit - middle aged men who have already had a heart attack - there is widespread disagreement about the reason for the benefit. Statins are weakly anti-inflammatory, and many ascribe any benefits entirely to this property, which they note can be better achieved in other ways.

Statins work by blocking an enzyme called HMG CoA Reductase, which is a long way upstream from the production of cholesterol. So the drugs have a large number of effects, since every branch product from that pathway is perturbed by statin administration, leaving the door wide open for a large number of effects (I struggle to call them side-effects, which happen when the drug affects a different target than the one intended), often in unpredictable ways. Cognitive decline and muscle dysfunction are commonly reported effects of statin use. Further, men using statins seem to have a slight reduction in the risk of prostate cancer, but women experience an increase in breast cancer risk. In both cases, the numbers are small enough that I would not make any decisions based on them.

So what is one to make of it all? The use of statins remains an unsettled issue. Independent verification of a pivotal result by an unbiased sponsor constitutes gold standard proof of something in science, and the ALLHAT-LL trial failed to find any benefit of statin use. Positive results have all come from trials where the sponsor had a direct stake in the outcome, and even those have never reported a survival benefit. We should not count on any more expensive statin trials in the future, since their patents have now expired, and the money has been drained from the system.

An important hallmark of cause and effect is a something like a linear relationship between the cause and the effect. In other words, the dose of the statin, the percentage cholesterol reduction, and the clinical benefit, should show a direct relationship. It may not be a perfect linear relationship, but some demonstrable dose-response should be observed. And if the cholesterol reduction is not meaningful, but the trial reports a meaningful result, then the better conclusion is that the benefit is from a different effect than cholesterol reduction.

With all the unanswered questions and objections, it is not possible to point to statins, and say, "There is proof that cholesterol reduction reduces the incidence of heart disease." And given all the other evidence inconsistent with the relationship between blood cholesterol and heart disease, no definitive conclusions are possible.

Finally, this discussion of statins is necessarily short, or it would change the character of this book. In addition to his book The Great Cholesterol Con, Malcolm Kendrick has written Doctoring Data, an exposé of many of the ways data are presented deceptively. I encourage everyone with more questions to read both.

Summary: The single independently-funded study on statins showed no benefit of any kind. Only those trials funded by pharmaceutical companies with a large stake in the outcome reported benefits. A long list of complaints against those reports undermines their credibility.

My Two Cents' Worth

Good against remotes is one thing. Good against a living, that's something else. ~ Han Solo

Star Wars purists will probably point out that I have that quote wrong. Solo probably said "good against *the* living..." as opposed to robots. I first saw Star Wars when I was 12, and for over forty years, understood Solo's meaning as, *tricks are amusing, but it's another thing entirely to survive and make a living.* My take has an important implication: If you had to bet real money on the true cause of heart disease, how would you decide who to believe? Would you rather trust someone who suffers no personal loss if they're wrong (the expert on a government committee), or someone who makes their living by betting on it, and would be wiped out entirely if they were wrong? I would side with the one who has skin in the game, every time. So who has the most skin in this game? I'd argue it is the life insurance industry. A life insurance policy is fundamentally a bet. It may be a hedge against other bets, such as a mortgage, but it remains a bet that you will die within a specified time frame, while they bet you won't die over that period. To make money, they need to issue more policies to people who will not die, yet pay their premiums. To get this right, they need to assess your risk of early death, and that requires a predictive measurement. Rest assured, they do not simply measure recommended blood lipids or cholesterol. That would have bankrupted them long ago. They have developed their own metrics, rooted in numerical facts.

The life insurance industry's favorite measure for the risk of an early death is gamma-glutamyl transferase (GGT), a marker of liver stress. Elevated GGT is highly predictive of cardiovascular and all-cause mortality (reviewed by Mason *et al.*, Preventive Cardiology 13:36-41, 2010, Koenig and Seneff, Disease Markers 818570, 2015).

Is it liver stress itself, or GGT in the blood, that causes the risk? If it were liver stress alone, then other markers of liver stress should show similar patterns, and GGT would not stand out like it does. And yet it stands out, suggesting it may be the risk factor, rather than merely a marker of the true risk factor. GGT is involved in the detoxification of reactive oxygen compounds in the liver. A liver over-stuffed with glucose is fighting elevated levels of reactive oxygen, so I would expect it to make more GGT. Some of those liver cells will die, releasing GGT into circulation. There, it can cause the very oxidation it is meant to protect against inside the cell. GGT is also found in atherosclerotic plaques, thus linking liver stress to atherosclerotic plaques, and plausibly, oxidized cholesterol. High GGT is also associated with diabetes, fatty liver disease, alcoholism, and systemic inflammation, which are all risk factors for heart disease.

On the strength of these observations, I suspect liver stress causes the release of GGT into the blood, which raises the risk of heart disease, and yet it is not the sole cause. I believe heart disease is really a number of different disorders whose only commonality is that they injure or kill heart tissue. When a person dies because their heart stopped, we rarely learn what actually happened inside the heart, so it is often reported as a heart attack, and assumed to have been caused by a ruptured plaque. That is only one of many ways to kill the heart, although it is thought to be the most common.

Earlier, I mentioned one possible mechanism of heart damage, involving the poisoning of the heart's mitochondria by trans fats that cannot be fully metabolized. Suddenly short of energy, those heart cells would rely on accelerated glycolysis to obtain what energy they can. The pyruvate that builds up cannot be converted to acetyl-CoA, because the poisoned mitochondria are unable to use it. So it is converted to lactic acid, which builds up and eventually poisons those heart muscle cells. The extent of damage would depend on how hard the heart was forced to work at that time, and whether certain regions of heart muscle were already weakened. Another way lactic acid can poison the heart is if the sympathetic nervous system loses regulation and burns out the heart. Cocaine is known to cause death by cardiac arrest, probably by the same mechanism. And of course, the classic plaque rupture and clot that blocks blood flow will also cause lactic acid buildup. On an optimistic note, when the body is burning fat because it lacks carbs, lactic acid buildup becomes improbable, since it is only generated by glucose metabolism.

To answer why diabetes raises the risk of the classic heart attack, we first need to understand how plaques build up in the first place. Sure, there's oxidized cholesterol inside them. But how does it get there, why does it happen at tightly localized spots in arteries but not veins, and why are clots of varying ages also in there, together with cellular debris?

Arterial Wounding: This model is introduced in Malcolm Kendrick's book, *The Great Cholesterol Con*. Rather than rely on lipoproteins burrowing through endothelium, he postulates something more plausible: The formation of an occasional wound on the endothelium of an artery. If endothelium is the equivalent of skin, then the wound would be the equivalent of a blister, or scrape. It might not look like either of those two, however. It might be a few endothelial cells getting ripped off their foundations by high-speed, turbulent blood flow. Veins are structurally similar to arteries, but do not develop plaques, which is telling. The speed at which blood flows through veins is slow. If it were a case of cholesterol coming out of suspension and settling down like sediment, it would happen where blood flows slowly, but it's the opposite. Further, plaques in arteries seem to form at places where the artery bends and kinks. Blood flow at those places will be turbulent, and one face of the inside of the artery will bear the brunt of the turbulence.

To an extent, wounding and healing are normal, and need not

lead to disease. A clot forms at the site of the wound, allowing for healing. But in contrast to clots on the exterior skin, or scabs, where healing happens under the scab, then the scab falls off, clots in arteries cannot be allowed to fall off. They would lodge into narrow blood vessels and block the flow of blood. Instead, a clot on the interior of the artery attracts all the raw materials needed to complete the repairs. Those raw materials include fat and cholesterol, that make up the membranes of every cell. Then, to prevent the clot from falling off, a new layer of endothelial cells overgrow the healing wound, and healing is completed under the new endothelium. If left undisturbed, the healing process is followed by the breakdown and cleanup of all the debris, and the artery wall is restored to working order. But until healing is complete, the material under the new endothelium is basically a plaque.

As mentioned several times, arterial plaques contain the remains of many clots of different ages, layered one on top of another. Integrated with them are the remnants of lipoproteins, the vesicles that carry fat and cholesterol. Instead of noticing only the remains of lipoproteins, we should notice multiple old clots, and also ask how they got there. The only possible explanation for multiple clots of different ages is a history of wounding that had not been fully cleaned up. Things get into the plaques when the wound is open, and are then stuck in there when new endothelium overgrows them.

If we further postulate that wounding happens repeatedly at high-risk locations such as kinks in an artery, there may not be sufficient time between events to heal and clean up all the debris. With many cycles of recurrent wounding, the plaque builds to ever greater proportions, until the last wound is simply too big for the artery. That final clot blocks the flow of blood, and a heart attack is the result.

I've mentioned oxidized cholesterol several times, and now it's time to marry it to the model of repeated wounding. Any explanation of how plaques form ultimately has to include an explanation for why oxidized cholesterol is in there. We now return to pattern B LDL, the old, sticky, dense, small particles that seem like they've been lost and forgotten. A significant proportion of the cholesterol in their core is oxidized. And when oxidized, cholesterol is prone to crystallization. That makes it very difficult to break up into morsels that can be easily taken up by cells, and removed from the system. If it's present in any appreciable amount, it will markedly slow the cleanup process. But high levels of GGT are also relevant, because GGT will get trapped in plaques, and further oxidize whatever cholesterol is trapped under the endothelium. These factors, working together, increase the amount of insoluble, oxidized cholesterol that is resistant to cleanup, and greatly increase the chances of another wound happening at the same place, adding to the size of the plaque. Any agent that adds to the oxidative stress or inflammation inside the plaque would make things worse. Below, another mechanism of plaque formation is introduced, involving inflammatory responses to infections. As I've said, I believe heart disease is an outcome, rather than a precise mechanism. Multiple causes are probable.

Other Contributors to Heart Disease:

Liver Stress: I've already covered GGT and liver stress, but so many arrows point in this direction that I suspect anything that raises liver stress will also raise heart disease risk. This begins with the fat cycle, where a liver starved of carbs does not accumulate fat, but instead imports what it needs from adipocytes. That person will have low triglycerides and high HDL, whereas the one with an excess of carbs will have high triglycerides and low HDL. Excessive consumption of alcohol raises triglycerides, causes liver fat accumulation, and elevated GGT. Fructose will do exactly the same as alcohol. A diabetic treated with drugs that stuff glucose into liver cells will probably make more GGT, to protect those cells from oxidative stress. But that GGT will leak into circulation, and cause general oxidative stress. How does the same protein protect from oxidative stress inside cells, yet cause oxidation in circulation? GGT transfers glutamyl groups reversibly, so if it's in a reducing environment such as the inside of a cell, it will keep the glutathione cycle going, to maintain that reducing environment. But in circulation, oxygen is more plentiful, and the process can work in reverse.

Oxidative Stress: When GGT and glutathione circulate through the blood together, they can cause oxidation of anything they come in contact with. This leads to destabilization of red blood cells, and leaking of their contents. Oxidation can liberate iron from proteins that keep it bound up, and free iron is like a wrecking ball in terms of the oxidative cascade it can unleash. Widespread oxidation can damage endothelium directly, and can accelerate the oxidation of cholesterol, especially if trapped in a healing arterial wound, otherwise known as a plaque. Oxidative stress can also damage all the organs of the body, and raises the risk of just about every disease of ageing, starting with those of the circulatory system.

Neurological Stress: Another factor known to play a role in heart disease is neurological stress, often simply called chronic stress. Malcolm Kendrick favors stress as the leading cause of heart disease. Acute stress as a trigger for a heart attack is not controversial. And chronic stress is also a known contributor to plaque formation. It appears that elevated stress increases the numbers of white blood cells that can cause inflammation. The stress response seems designed to prepare us to confront trouble, where a wound and infection can be the result. But when stress is chronic, and there is no wound, those white blood cells go off looking for trouble. They often find it in arterial plaques, which are sites of previous wounds. The white blood cells inflame those plaques, and make them prone to rupture (http://www.sciencemag.org/news/2014/06/how-stress-can-clog-your-arteries).

So why is stress not the leading theory? The medical establishment is not comfortable with the idea of stress, because there is no numerical measure associated with it. It is much easier to measure LDL in the blood than to take the time to get to know the patient, and look for the telltale signs of chronic stress. The hormone cortisol is a mediator of stress, but it undergoes substantial natural fluctuations, so no single measurement can paint an accurate picture of chronic stress. However, chronically elevated cortisol also stimulates gluconeogenesis (conversion of proteins to glucose). This is accompanied by elevated VLDL, elevated triglycerides, lower HDL, and elevated clotting factors, including fibrinogen. Exactly what we think of as risk factors for heart disease.

Inflammation: Chronic inflammation caused by stress is a known risk factor for heart disease, and diabetes is a very inflammatory disease. Everything from the advanced glycation end-products that arise from the reaction of glucose with the body's proteins, to the damage to the microvasculature, increases overall inflammation. The white blood cells responsible for inflammation then invade arterial plaques, and destabilize them. Dr. Uffe Ravnskov, who deserves more credit than I've managed to give him, considers inflammation due to infection to be a leading contributor to heart disease. For instance, the bacteria that cause periodontal infections are often found in arterial plaques. Infections of those plaques could lead to their invasion by white blood cells, destabilization of the plaque, and rupture. It's not hard to imagine several factors working together, to increase the risk of heart disease.

Insulin and Blood Pressure. Type II diabetics have too much insulin. Carb-fed people without blood glucose abnormalities may also have too much insulin, and high blood pressure. First, insulin causes fluid retention by the kidneys, increasing blood volume. Second, insulin stimulates the smooth muscle cells around arteries to grow stronger, and squeeze harder. This further raises blood pressure, and stiffens the arteries. They used to say age stiffens arteries, or maybe they still do. Or cholesterol. But cholesterol does not line the length of an artery, like grease lines drains. The biggest factor in the stiffening of arteries is the squeeze from the smooth muscles wrapping those arteries. It's easy to imagine how high blood pressure could cause hemorrhagic strokes, where small blood vessels simply burst open. But how can it contribute to plaque formation, rupture, and clotting associated with heart disease?

To help with that, imagine this scenario, that seems to happen to me all too often. A large bird defecates on your car's windshield, and when you try to wipe it with your windshield wipers and wiper fluid, you soon find it spread over the entire windshield. It's worse than ever. So you get out of the car, and go for the garden hose. But it has no spray nozzle attached, and letting the water pour out the end does not provide enough pressure to clean your windshield. So you squeeze it with your thumb, and force the water out a much smaller hole, to increase the pressure. This increases the speed of the water, and soon cleans your car windshield. Lesson: By forcing the water to come out a smaller hole, the speed of the water went way up, and dislodged things that were stuck before.

Similarly, by forcing blood to travel through an artery that does not flex with each pulse, the speed of the blood is far faster. At bends and kinks in the artery, the addition of turbulence to the flow can scour the wall of the artery with unusually high shear forces. This leads to wounds, and even sloughing off of endothelial cells, like a scrape on skin. This can led to repeated wounding at that same place, and the formation of an arterial plaque.

Glucose and ECM Damage. Glycation of extracellular matrix proteins by excess glucose damages their ability to support endothelial cells. This weakens the ability of the endothelial cell to grip its foundation, and lowers the threshold for the cell to be ripped away. This is compounded by the direct damage excess glucose inflicts on endothelial cells, by over-stimulating the glucosamine pathway, as those cells have particular difficulty coping with that pathway. So the endothelial cells are weakened, and sick, plus they are attached to a matrix that does not provide as much support as it used to, as a result of glycation. However, treating diabetes with drugs that control blood glucose does not improve heart disease risk, so ECM damage alone is probably not a principal causal factor.

Summary: A more plausible model for the development of heart disease is repeated wounding of the lining of arteries, at places of high velocity, turbulent blood flow. Wounds heal, but the next wound happens before healing and cleanup are finished. Oxidized cholesterol is a lot harder to clean up, so cleanup is much slower, and chances increase that it won't have healed before the next wound happens. Diabetes increases blood pressure, making wounds more frequent. It increases oxidative stress, worsening the damage to the endothelium, and the supply of oxidized cholesterol. Finally, diabetes treatment strategies increase the supply of pattern B LDL, the form most susceptible to oxidation of its cholesterol cargo.

PART TWO: Walking the Other Path

Chapter 5: The Realization

The ideal of medicine is to eliminate the need of a physician. ~ William J. Mayo

I was visiting my father, a retired physician. Seeing a dressing on my toe one morning, he did not ask about the wound. Instead, his words were, "I need to measure your blood glucose." I knew right away what he was getting at. To be perfectly honest, I already knew I must be diabetic, but managed to avoid confronting it. With the reading of 325 mg/dl, the truth was finally out in the open. But how did I get here? I had always been athletic, and had only become moderately overweight, when actual body fat is considered. Traditional body mass index (BMI) measurements would by then classify me as obese, but I'm muscular, and the BMI does not normalize for that. At over six feet tall, I wore pants with a 36 inch waist for most of my adult life, which had expanded to a snug 38 in the previous five or ten years.

I had been active in sports for most of my life, although I was never truly slim. I was most passionate about hockey, and played as a goaltender, well into my forties. When playing goal, you spend much of your time crouched low, with your knees bent, always ready to quickly push off in either direction. And my legs were, and still are, very muscular. I could produce bursts of power from them, but I never had true endurance. I always needed breaks to catch my breath, and clear the lactic acid from my legs. In retrospect, I was fermenting glucose, and not getting a lot of aerobic exercise. I was never good at running distances, and even when in otherwise good shape, long hikes quickly tired me out.

I recall that when playing hockey, as early as my thirties, I began to feel like my energy was sagging. I would feel a little lightheaded, and there would be a tingling sensation in my fingertips, and eyelids. I decided it was probably low blood glucose, so to compensate, I did the worst thing possible. I used to keep a water bottle on the top of the net, and take drinks during stoppages in play. But to combat my low energy, I switched from water to a sports drink, to keep my energy levels up. It never crossed my mind that half the calories in the drink were in the form of fructose, which would do nothing to boost my energy, but would overtax my liver. In retrospect, this would have been a good time to check my insulin levels. My blood glucose would likely have been normal at that time, or close to normal. But my insulin would probably be chronically elevated, a hallmark of insulin resistance. Instead, I assured myself that since it felt like my glucose was low, not high, it could not be the start of diabetes. It was something else, and there was no need to concern myself with it. After all, the symptoms of diabetes should be what I might feel after dinner, if I had eaten a large plate of pasta or rice.

As I graduated from youth into middle age, life got very busy. Like most people, my time for exercise was limited, as was anything outside my commitments to family and work. Eventually, I put on some weight. A typical supper at my house consisted of vegetables, lean meat, some sort of sauce, and a plate full of rice, or potatoes, or other forms of carbohydrate, to *top me up*. As a family, we designed our meals this way to conform with what we knew about public health guidelines, or the *Food Pyramid*. Afraid to eat too much fat, we knew we had to fill ourselves somehow, so after satisfying our nutrient needs with vegetables and lean meat, we finished filling ourselves with what we (then) believed to be the least harmful food group: Carbs.

Generally, my wife and I made an effort to favor unsaturated fats over saturated fats, because we were told that saturated fat could lead to heart disease. I never knew where this advice came from, and it never occurred to me to question it. Eventually, I began to hear about *trans fat* being very bad for cardiovascular health, despite being unsaturated. I was taken aback when I realized I had been eating it, thinking it was good. I could have questioned whether the whole saturated versus unsaturated fat paradigm might also be wrong, but I did not. But I wondered, in passing, how the official advice could have been so wrong, for so long. All the same, I went along with the new recommendations without further questions. I was too busy to worry about my health.

I had other symptoms that should have alerted me to my escalating insulin resistance, including increased sweating. I also became chronically thirsty, and would drink copious amounts of water, then pass it as very dilute urine. I would occasionally register elevated blood pressure when donating blood. But not much was made of it, and I dismissed it as *probably too much coffee.* Whatever the symptom, I always found a reason to avoid admitting the facts to myself.

If you're asking whether the above lapses are indicative of my critical thinking skills, I understand. I won't pretend to have been better than I was. I suspect nobody will reach middle age and develop diabetes, without having had a few indications along the way that things were not going swimmingly well. And if you're like me, you might wonder if it's your fault. I did. And that sense of shame had a lot to do with why I did not want to confront it. Had I known how easy it was to change the course of the disease, I certainly would have. But where would I have learned that, in retrospect? Advice from the American Diabetes Association would only make things worse, but you have to reach a certain threshold of suspicion before you start to scrutinize an organization like that. That suspicion only came much later.

Eventually, I recognized that my fitness had slipped too far. I stopped playing hockey in my forties, but I did not replace it with other forms of exercise. I had every reason to suspect my blood pressure was high, and I was not regulating my blood glucose effectively. I began to worry about the implications for my cardiac health, but not enough to get a complete physical. I had recently undergone tests for a life insurance policy. Surely they would have alerted me if there were any serious problems. I was in denial, but I convinced myself to take precautions. I bought an elliptical orbiter, and began to exercise regularly. This helped me lose a little weight, and rebuild some cardiovascular fitness. If I ate a carb-heavy meal, and felt uncomfortable as my glucose spiked, I had the impression that exercise helped ease the discomfort. I knew there was a problem with my health, but I could not bring myself to confront it. *Sure, I'll deal with it, some time soon.*

The skin on my toes had become thick, and would occasionally split. Healing was very slow, as the wound would split anew whenever walked upon. I went to shaving the skin down with a utility razor, which helped any cracks heal properly. But one time, I went a little too deep, and caused a small wound, less than a quarter inch across, and approximately round in shape. It was only just through the skin, and it drew very little blood. I treated it as best I could, and changed the dressing regularly, but it refused to heal. It slowly became an ulcer.

At that point, I could not deny I had diabetes. Impaired circulation in the toes, resulting in poor wound healing, is a hallmark of the disease. That was when I paid that visit to my father, and had my blood glucose measured for the first time. He made several additional measurements over the following days, more for my benefit than his, and confirmed the numbers. I say it was for my benefit, because he knew I was diabetic with the first measurement, if not when he first saw my toe. But he also understood the need to persuade me of it. He then gave me a small shot of insulin, which he had been taking for a few years, as the course of his own type II diabetes had reached the insulin-dependent stage. He measured my glucose again, and seeing little change, declared it to be insulin resistant. He also insisted I get a referral to see an endocrinologist, who would get me the right combination of drugs to treat my diabetes. To drive the point home, he called my wife, and made her promise to make me see a doctor, and not try to treat it myself. He knew my nature would compel me to question everything.

After that first measurement, I abruptly refused to consume anything with so much as a trace of carbohydrate. It was as if all the anxiety and denial about my health had suddenly been focused on the enemy, now in the open: Glucose. The last beer I ever drank was the previous day, and I declined anything sweet. Dad eventually became a little frustrated with my attitude, when he offered me a sweet muffin, and I visibly shuddered in response.

"It's not normal for diabetics to stop eating carbohydrates," he objected.

"Well, shouldn't it be?" There was no answer, so I added, "You want me to take a combination of drugs, so I can continue to eat sugar and carbs?"

"That's how the disease is treated."

We changed the subject, but at an instinctive level, I was sure of myself. The disease was not being treated correctly. *Rather than take both poison and a marginal antidote, is it not better to stop poisoning yourself in the first place?* In keeping with my nature, I was already scheming as to how I could satisfy dad's demands, at least in spirit, while finding an alternative to multiple medications.

Of course, there was another problem. Glucose was the body's principal energy source. Everything I had been taught spoke to this. Plants use photosynthesis to make glucose, and respiration reverses the process, to make energy. How could you live without glucose?

My instinctive aversion to anything containing sugar or starch was now in conflict with years of education. It was time to question everything. Over the years, I'd occasionally been exposed to Eastern schools of medical thought, which now loomed larger than ever before. In principle, there's no disputing Eastern concepts such as considering overall health in the context of nutrition and lifestyle. I also knew the Western medical system's reliance on targeted intervention was oversold, and provided no incentive to solve a health problem with a change in lifestyle or nutrition. But to me, the knock on Eastern thinking was that it sounded too vague, and rarely provided any specific recommendations.

I knew the importance of nutrition was underappreciated. I had once heard it stated as, "Bad nutrition, and medicine can't help. Good nutrition, and medicine is unnecessary." That felt then, and it still does today, like the overstatement of a valid concept. Antibiotics have saved billions of lives, after all. But I was facing a concrete problem, and needed a concrete answer: Could nutrition break the back of diabetes?

I was superficially familiar with low carbohydrate diets for weight loss, but it turns out I knew few details. I assumed they consisted of lean meats and vegetables, and worried they would leave me hungry. Diets that leave you hungry fail with 100% certainty. Nevertheless, as I stumbled along, I remained firm in my resolve to stop eating any carb-rich foods, switching instead to vegetables and protein. The jolt of being ripped out of my denial caused me some significant stomach discomfort at first, so I did not initially experience cravings. That helped offset some of the mistakes I made early in my recovery.

Summary: Diabetes was a long time in the making, and I wanted to break it the first day I was aware of it. Avoiding carbs was an instinctive reaction, before I knew the details of how it all worked. I was made aware from the start that it was not the normal way diabetes was treated. My reaction was, "Shouldn't it be?"

Chapter 6: The First Few Weeks

Poisons and medicine are oftentimes the same substance given with different intents. ~ Peter Mere Latham

Once I realized the nature of the monster inside me, I wanted to purge it *immediately*, if not sooner. I didn't know what I was doing, and I didn't know the extent of the damage I had done to my health. I also didn't understand all the particulars of the diet I was now embracing by default. But the details could wait. Getting my glucose down was suddenly my all-consuming priority.

Five days elapsed between my first measurement at 325 mg/dl, and my returning home. As soon as I returned, I went to the drug store to buy a glucose meter and test strips. Returning from the drug store, I measured a fasting 229 mg/dl at 11:30 on a Saturday morning, which was far better than the previous week, while I was traveling. I had been doing my best to avoid all carbs, even if I was probably eating too much protein at the time. I never entertained the thought that a hundred point reduction in five days was something to be happy about. 229 mg/dl was still far too high. All I thought about was how much farther there was to go, and whether it would even be achievable.

That evening, my wife and I had some wine, to acknowledge my return home, and to release the tension of the past week or so. The following morning, a Saturday, I measured 275 mg/dl, with a headache. This was a turn in the wrong direction (or a measurement error. I did not measure such high glucose levels for very long, so I can't be sure what kind of variation is to be expected when blood glucose is that high). At the time, I didn't appreciate that getting glucose out of circulation was far from the only concern. I simply wanted to be rid of it, and felt I had to do something to start bringing it down aggressively. I had not yet found a doctor, so I could not access prescription drugs, and in any case did not want to use them over the long run. My choice in the short term: Supplements.

I chose supplements because of a report that intrigued me back in the 1990s. When the insulin receptor is activated, it is subsequently turned off by the action of protein tyrosine phosphatase-1B (PTP-1B), and insulin resistance is associated with, among other things, more PTP-1B in affected cells. So if you could turn off PTP-1B, you could lessen insulin resistance, and potentiate the insulin signal. And I remembered that a component of cinnamon was able to block PTP-1B activity. Before doing any more reading, and furious with my 275 mg/dl reading that morning, I went straight to the drug store, and bought cinnamon supplement capsules, promptly taking one. By noon, I was down to 225 mg/dl, a drop of 50 points in a few hours. Later that day, I measured under 200 mg/dl, and never again measured over 250 mg/dl. That day, I took several additional measurements which came in between 182 and 225 mg/dl. *Wow, supplements can make a difference*, I thought.

I soon found a report stating that while cinnamon works as advertised, over the long-term, it could be toxic to the liver. What to do? It turns out that true cinnamon, which is not considered toxic, comes only from Ceylon (Sri Lanka), and is expensive. So much so that hardly anyone uses it. *Cassia* is a related tree, that is used in nearly every cinnamon prep I came across (I later found true Ceylon cinnamon at Costco). Cassia contains a compound called coumarin, which is the source of the toxicity. But there was a solution. Coumarin is fat-soluble, while the PTP-1B inhibitor(s) are water soluble. Cinnamon extracts that have only the water-soluble components offer the pharmacologically active ingredient, but not the toxic one. I saw one at Costco called Cinsulin, and I had a one from Swanson called Cinnulin. Both names imply what it's used for, and it appeared to work, while I was insulin resistant. It eventually stops working to lower glucose levels, once insulin resistance is broken (you don't need to overcome what's no longer there).

In retrospect, while cinnamon works to overcome insulin resistance, even the water-extracts lacking coumarin have the potential to stress the liver. They are, after all, undermining the liver's innate defenses against taking up too much glucose. I now wonder how much of the alleged toxicity of cinnamon is actually attributable to excess glucose uptake by the livers of diabetics, who take large doses of cinnamon under the assumption they're treating their disease.

I was now reliably measuring under 200 mg/dl, and strictly avoiding carbs. Having had success with one supplement, I started to wonder about others. What followed was an extensive search, and I started to experiment with many different supplements. Gymnema

Sylvestre has long been used in Indian medicine to lower blood glucose, so I added it. Korean Ginseng, Astragalus root, alpha-lipoic Acid, and corisolic acid were others I added to my regimen, at least for a time. If you're thinking, *he's overdoing it*, you're one step ahead of where I was at the time. I was impatient to get my glucose down, because I imagined it like the poison it was, rotting me away from the inside.

By the time I found a doctor and had my blood tested, two weeks into my recovery, my glucose was down to 160 mg/dl. However, my doctor observed that my HbA1C was 10.9%. This value was predictive of glucose in the 250 mg/dl range, and I knew from my frequent measurements that my glucose had been well below 250 mg/dl for about the previous ten days or so. The HbA1C test assumes a relatively stable glucose level, and when in rapid flux, recent changes have an outsized impact. So it's probable that my HbA1C before I started my carb boycott might have been appreciably higher. If my average blood glucose was in the range of the 325 mg/dl of my first measurement, then my HbA1C would have been about 13%. Bottom line, I had now cut my blood glucose in half in two weeks, without drugs. Good start? Well, yes, and no.

I had not yet mastered low-carb dieting, so I was ripe for some mistakes. One day, I decided to fry some cauliflower, which I knew to be low in carbs, but I breaded it, because I did not think a few bread crumbs could contribute so many carbs. I then measured 243 mg/dl, a definite setback. But I took extra Cinsulin, and by that evening, two hours after dinner, I was back down at 163 mg/dl.

The following day at 11:30 am, on an empty stomach, I measured 207 mg/dl. That was frustrating, but I attributed it to the lingering effects of the breaded cauliflower. Fortunately, that was the last reading I ever had above 200 mg/dl. In another two days, I was regularly measuring below 150 mg/dl, but a curious thing was also happening. Irrespective of whether I was fasting or eating breakfast, my blood glucose would rise between my 7:30 measurement, when I got up, and one I made at 11:30, before lunch. It was by as much as twenty points, and it would drop by twenty to thirty points several hours after a meal. I explained to myself that my liver was making glucose while I was fasting, because it was used to a high level in my blood, but my cells took up glucose after a meal, while the meal itself did not provide any. I was probably making too much glucagon, a hormone secreted by the alpha cells of the pancreas, that tells the liver to make glucose out of protein. Alpha cells become insulin resistant in diabetes, and had not yet reverted to their post-diabetic state.

By day seventeen, any glucose reading above 150 mg/dl was the exception, and my daily averages were under 140 mg/dl. I felt some satisfaction at how far I had come, and how fast, but I was now confronting another health issue. It had probably been there all along, but I was only now becoming aware of it, and it got a little dicey with me for a while.

Summary: Supplements can bring down blood glucose, like drugs can. But what happens to the glucose after being taken up by cells? That's an important consideration.

Blood Pressure

Several points need to preface what I will share about my experiences. First, low carb diets are widely acclaimed for reducing blood pressure, as lower insulin levels result in less fluid retention, leading to naturally reduced blood pressure. In fact, some detractors of such diets for weight loss claim that the rapid weight loss is entirely due to fluid loss. When I hear that accusation, I conclude that the diet is indisputably effective at reversing excessive fluid retention. And the feedback I received from several people I converted to the diet confirms that their blood pressure came down dramatically, within about two weeks. All reported blood pressure drops of twenty to thirty points (systolic), whereupon they discontinued their medications. But alas, type II diabetics will need to be a lot more patient, and we'll cover that point a little later.

The second point is that men with muscular arms register higher blood pressure than their thinner counterparts. Blood pressure is defined as the pressure required by that inflatable cuff to squeeze the arm at the bicep enough to stop the flow of arterial blood. As such, it has to squeeze through muscle, to reach the artery. They always tell you to relax your arm, because they know that tensing it would fight the force of the cuff. But simply having more muscle mass on the bicep forces the cuff to squeeze through extra layers. Lastly, I discovered I have a severe case of *white coat syndrome*. That's what doctors call it when blood pressure, and pulse, shoot up dramatically exactly when being measured. I experience immediate anxiety when I hear that Velcro on the cuff being pried apart, ready to strangle my arm. Even as I was editing this manuscript, I would become tense when re-reading the preceding sentence for the tenth time, or so. At home, I would find it necessary to put the cuff on, then relax for fifteen minutes or so, before I could get a good measurement. At the doctor's office, the nurse charges into the room, and aggressively does the measurement, frowning the whole time. I don't have a chance. All in all, I'm confident that the act of measuring my blood pressure is bad for my health. But of course, I did not know any of this at the time.

I expected to find my blood pressure elevated, but the first time it was measured, it registered 160/110. By waiting in the examination room until I had calmed a bit, we could get it down to about 150/100. It is uncertain whether that was still artificially elevated due to anxiety. Nonetheless, the doctor suggested in a persuasively understated manner that it would be *really good* to bring that down, sooner rather than later. We agreed that as my fitness improved, and my weight came down, it would also bring down my blood pressure, but in the meantime, it would be best to start some medication. She started me on lisinopril, an inhibitor of angiotensin converting enzyme, which blocks one pathway to high blood pressure. But that's where things became complicated.

At around the same time, I started numerous supplements to bring down my glucose, and something went wrong soon after I started lisinopril. It's not possible to say what caused it, but my blood pressure spiked. I measured over 180/115 for several days. And whereas I had previously exercised strenuously with little difficulty, I was now dizzy. I couldn't get my heart rate up to support my energy consumption, and could not exercise. I felt terrible. I called my doctor, who added a diuretic to my medications. A *water-pill*, it made my kidneys excrete excess water, hoping that by lowering the volume of my blood, it would lower the pressure. It failed to help, and it produced awful side effects. My blood pressure was now at the edge of where you might be best advised to check in to the emergency room and have the full complement of machines hooked up.

I was close to panic at this point. My blood pressure might have been high all along, but before, I could at least exercise. Now, after beginning medications, it was worse than ever, and it made me feel awful. Finally, my wife said, "You know, you've added so many supplements, it's really impossible to pin it on any one thing." Struck by my stupidity, I stopped all my supplements immediately. By the time I returned to see the doctor, a few days later, my blood pressure had receded somewhat, to about the 160/110 range (measured by that frowning nurse) of before everything went bad. She did an electrocardiogram, confirmed that my heart was healthy, and replaced my blood pressure meds with Bystolic, a new inhibitor of the beta adrenergic receptor, otherwise known as a beta blocker. Adrenaline raises blood pressure when the body needs to do something athletic, or often times when it's stressed. If the adrenaline response is always active, blood pressure can be always high. Bystolic blocks that response. Fortunately, it worked, and quickly got my blood pressure below 150/100. But where was the promised blood pressure reduction from the low carb diet? I had lost weight, and my fitness was constantly improving, but my blood pressure was essentially the same as when I had started. Could I be some kind of mutant? I searched furiously for any report that might suggest such diets could fail to improve the blood pressure of certain people, but found nothing. Every report lauded the diet for reducing blood pressure.

Next, I started reconsidering all my supplements. There are sporadic reports of Gymnema Sylvestre raising blood pressure, so I eliminated it. Likewise for Korean Ginseng. I started adding the other supplements back to my regimen, and soon after I resumed Astragalus, my blood pressure again spiked over 160. I stopped it, and within a few days, it returned to my previous readings. Researching it, at first it seemed that Astragalus should lower blood pressure. Eventually, however, I found obscure references to it raising blood pressure. If that level of uncertainty is to be expected for supplements, where nobody has poured billions into characterizing all the possible complications, I should add that lisinopril is not to be presumed innocent, either. There was one report out of Albert Einstein Medical School suggesting that patients with low renin levels experienced elevated blood pressure on lisinopril. Renin is made by the kidneys, and is a blood pressure regulator. My renin was never tested, so I don't know if that describes me, or not.

There's a lesson in my early experiences. I was impatient to fix years of neglect in only a few weeks, and before I even knew how bad things really were. I changed too much at once, so when it went wrong, I could not quickly identify what I needed to correct, or even have a baseline to compare against. If I'm honest about it, my attitude at the time mirrored that of the medical system: Anything that reduces blood glucose and blood pressure is good, and that's all there is to it. I lost sight of the fact, or never saw it in the first place, that overall health is the primary objective, and other metrics are only signposts along the way.

My blood pressure came down slowly, and it took more than six months before I could confidently discontinue my medication. Why the difference between me, and so many others who saw immediate improvement on a low carb diet?

Being diabetic, I had extensive damage to my microvasculature. The consequences are that there is less space into which the circulatory system can pump blood. That creates more back-pressure, and higher blood pressure. The timing of when my blood pressure finally came down seemed to coincide with the original ulcer on my toe finally healing over, which suggests the recovery of my microvasculature may have been a limiting factor. But there were other factors, too. Those years of excess insulin would have made the smooth muscle cells wrapping my arteries extra thick, and inflexible. Every time the heart pumps, the lack of *give* in the arteries produces an elevated systolic pressure.

The combination of damaged microvasculature and rigid arteries were probably the driving forces in raising my blood pressure to such dangerous levels. And while my insulin surely came down dramatically in the first three weeks, it would take much longer for the smooth muscle cells wrapping my arteries to revert to a normal level of tone.

When I did not quickly see the results I was expecting, there was a substantial temptation to give up, and simply go on the pharmacological regimen of drugs, while eating the low-fat, high carb recommended diet. And now that I understand why my body reacted as it did, I can predict that other diabetics who try low carb dieting will also find that their blood pressure does not improve as quickly as it does for others.

In retrospect, I've come to see blood pressure from a different perspective. If arteries are narrowed, blood pressure increases to maintain the flow rate through those arteries. If blood pressure is reduced by a drug, it will reduce blood flow, just like turning a tap half way to *off* will reduce water flow. So if the kidneys require a certain flow rate to effectively filter blood, won't reducing it compromise the function of the kidney? If the body's tissues get less blood flow, won't they suffer various effects? I've found different perspectives on the question. Medical authorities in Germany are far more concerned whether the heart is strong enough to facilitate sufficient blood flow than they are about blood pressure. High blood pressure would seem to be an indicator of a problem with the cardiovascular system, rather than being the problem itself. And artificially reducing blood pressure is like reducing a fever without fighting the infection behind it.

Malcolm Kendrick has written that he does not know his own blood pressure, and doesn't care. He cites studies of blood pressure reduction that do nothing to improve overall mortality. I've come closer to his position, as I've gained confidence in my cardiovascular fitness. The fact that I had to deal with these issues at precisely the same time as I was adjusting my metabolism from burning carbs to fats made everything far more complicated, and frightening, than it probably needed to be.

Summary: My blood pressure spiked after starting supplements and blood pressure meds. I started too many new things at once. Even after I fixed those, my blood pressure took a good six months to come down, far slower than advertised on the high fat low carb diet. Diabetics will require extra time to see the benefits. Too much insulin for so long would have stiffened my artery muscles, while damage to small blood vessels took time to heal.

Weight Loss

The second day of a diet is always easier than the first. By the second day you're off it. ~ Jackie Gleason

I was recently informed that Kim Kardashian announced she had lost 75 pounds on a ketogenic diet. This one news item will undoubtedly raise the public profile of the diet much more than science ever could. But news of celebrity diets is not the most trustworthy. For starters, I have yet to find a celebrity who admits their diet was assisted by liposuction. And any details of the diet will be vetted by their PR guys, who might not allow any mention of lots of animal fat.

Nevertheless, it is a given that weight loss goes hand in hand with an improvement in blood glucose levels, blood pressure, and blood lipids. So every time a diabetic goes to the doctor, he/she will reliably be told, *lose weight, and your symptoms will improve.* Of course, *how* you are supposed to lose weight is never mentioned, because if there's one thing doctors know from experience, it's that diets don't work. Even when they *do* work, they only work temporarily. Medical wisdom says that if you ask any dieter a year or two later if they are still on the diet, the answer will be *no.* Most diets are not sustainable, because they leave you hungry. And even with the precedent of the Atkins diet, the notion that diets can have a lasting impact is simply too far outside most medical professionals' comfort zones. So they revert to the standard advice they know will not make any trouble for them: "Eat less, exercise more, and enter into negative caloric storage. You will lose weight, and your other metrics will also improve." Implicit in this advice is that obesity and diabetes are a result of your personal failings. In short, *you eat too much, and you sit on your duff too much.*

A longstanding argument continues to play out between those who hold that weight loss is about having enough discipline to eat less and exercise more (the quality of the person), and those who hold that appetite and energy are highly regulated processes, and all you need to do is hack the regulatory mechanisms (the quality of the diet/environment). Proponents of the energy balance paradigm, who always seem to be effortlessly thin, will cite the first law of thermodynamics as irrefutable proof. Those who disagree are said to be ignorant of Newton's laws. I'll be the first to admit, molecular biology does not require much rigor in physics, but I'm not ignorant of Newton's laws. My specialty is in the mechanisms by which biological processes are regulated, and by extension, that includes appetite and energy. So without disputing Isaac Newton, I would rather ask *why* a person eats too much, or exercises too little. Why, in response to exercising more, does he eat more. Or why in response to eating less, she has no energy for exercise. Once framed that way, and looking at the signals the body has to work with, it is no longer a matter of gluttony or sloth, and the types of calories consumed make all the difference.

The primary focus of this book is diabetes, and for me, weight loss was an added bonus. By contrast, most of the literature on ketogenic dieting is centered around weight loss, with the other health benefits being added bonuses. But the two are interlinked, and in reducing my blood glucose, weight loss was automatic.

One widely acknowledged reason why it is not accurate to say that every calorie is equal is because not all are absorbed with the same efficiency. Carbohydrates tend to be absorbed in their entirety, since they are water soluble, and are easily broken down into simple sugars that are readily absorbed. By contrast, fats are not water soluble, so absorbing them is dependent on additional factors. One is the presence of bile, produced by the liver and secreted into the small intestine. It acts like dish detergent, to break up the droplets of fat and allow their uptake in the small intestine. Do you want to guess what factor stimulates the release of bile from the gall bladder? Bonus points if you guessed insulin. The body will not absorb more fat than it can handle at any given time, and insulin prepares it to handle more. After all, if insulin is circulating, so is glucose, which is going to be needed by fat cells, to store dietary fat.

Likewise, if insulin is not active, fat cannot be stored, appetite drops, dietary fats quickly satisfy hunger, bile secretion drops, and over time, as fat cells run low on glycerol, they release fat for use as energy.

In the seasonal glucose feast scenario, carbohydrate abundance stimulates the buildup of as much fat as possible, but the key is that the feast ends after a few weeks. As the carbohydrates disappear, insulin levels drop, all remaining liver fat is finally packaged up and sent to fat cells, the muscles regain their insulin sensitivity, and equilibrium is restored. After a short transition, fats are again mobilized and burned, and the person regains their physical energy, which will be needed for hunting, and bringing home the occasional winter meal of protein and fat.

The problem is that what worked perfectly well when famine followed feast, does not work when feast follows feast follows feast, indefinitely. The insulin-driven fat-building response continues to build on itself, in order to build up as much fat as possible, while the feast is available. Hunger begets eating and fat building, insulin resistance, and more hunger. That same process is hard-wired into our genetic programming, which has not changed simply because we have constant access to sugar and refined carbohydrates. The result is that fructose is always overloading the liver, and fat is always being built up. The only way to break the cycle is to starve the insulin response of its fuel, as we would have in ancient times.

Viewed this way, it becomes clear why the gaining or losing of weight is not as simple as calories in, versus calories out. Yes, the calories are consumed, and are not burned, but the body's innate programs regulate everything, and those programs have not received the memo that we no longer live as hunter/gatherers.

The first month on a ketogenic diet is typically when weight melts off the body, like soap lather rinsing off in the shower. I exercised regularly, which helped, but the rate of weight loss was staggering. I was losing weight at something like a pound a day. At my next doctor's appointment, she was suddenly worried that something serious had gone wrong with my health, because of the speed at which I was losing weight. My clothes were hanging off me, loosely, where they had been snug only two weeks ago. I had to assure her that I had been exercising at least one hour per day, in my rush to drop my glucose levels. Surely I could not sustain that kind of pace if there was something seriously wrong. She accepted the explanation, but I don't think she had any idea what was going on with me.

Part of the initial weight loss was the depletion of my glycogen reserves, and loss of the extra water that comes with it. Even more water loss came when my insulin levels dropped down from their very high, type-II diabetic levels, reversing the kidney's water retention. But there was fat loss, also. That was obvious when looking in the mirror. I went from wearing pants with a 38-inch waist, and feeling tight, to being able to take them off without unbuttoning. In no time, size 36 again fit very comfortably. Then, after a drop of about 40 pounds in six weeks, I abruptly stopped losing weight. My fitness was constantly improving, my stomach was nearly flat, and my weight flat lined. The body knows better than to allow itself to become emaciated, when it is properly nourished. Is that a good thing, or should I wish my equilibrium weight was lower?

One often sees the body mass index (BMI) used as a measurement of obesity. Perhaps you would be surprised to learn that using the BMI charts, nearly all professional athletes would be classed overweight, or even obese. And I'm not talking about NFL linemen who need supplemental oxygen between plays. I'm talking about Olympic sprinters, NHL hockey players, and others who, if you met them at the beach, you'd marvel at their fitness. My BMI now comes in at exactly 30, the boundary between overweight and class I obese. That's with a flat stomach, and when I look in the mirror, I'm happy with what I see. But surely, there must be data showing it's better to have a lower BMI, right? That is another example of a bias that was gradually accepted as fact, but is not true.

One study looked at BMI versus all-cause mortality (Flegal et al., 2005. JAMA 293:1861-7). And the publication serves as a warning about not trusting the title, which says that being overweight causes extra mortality. But the data in the paper clearly show that the *overweight* (BMI between 25 and 30) have the *lowest* overall mortality. Obese class I (BMI between 30 and 35) are a close second. Suddenly, I don't feel so bad sitting on the border between the two. Third are those whose weight is considered normal (BMI 18.5 to 25). The two tails of the chart, *obese class II* and *underweight*, have the highest rates of mortality. Which of those would you guess is more dangerous? And the loser is ... underweight. Those with a BMI of less than 18.5 have the highest overall mortality rate, even higher than those considered class II obese, with a BMI over 35. Consequently, I don't give BMI any credence. With a glance, any doctor can tell who needs to lose weight, and who does not.

Summary: Insulin causes fat buildup. Once insulin levels drop, energy levels rise, appetite is controlled, and fat can be burned off. Loss of excess weight is inevitable. But it stabilizes very quickly, once equilibrium is reached.

Sugar

Refined sugar is probably the single worst thing for anyone to consume, and is now banned at my house. As is anything sweetened with sugar. And it is important not to be fooled by ingredient lists. Sugar has 56 names, and counting. Adding the word *organic* changes nothing. *No sugar added* only means there's plenty already there, so they didn't need to add more. *But I have a sweet tooth*, some will say. Fear not. There are alternatives. And I'm not talking about products of the chemical industry, such as saccharine, aspartame, acesulfame, sucralose, etc. Those don't taste good to begin with, and who knows about their health consequences. I'm talking about truly excellent alternatives.

Most people know about stevia. It has an extremely sweet taste, so a very small amount goes a long way. It is usually blended with something else, to bring it down to a useful potency. But stevia may not be the best choice. Trace amounts are fine, but in higher amounts, it tastes bitter. Also, stevia does not add bulk to food, the way sugar does.

Erythritol is commonly used to dilute stevia. It can form crystals just like regular sugar, and add bulk to food. It is a natural product, non-caloric, and that fraction that is absorbed is quickly excreted in urine. Erythritol is about 70% as sweet as sugar, and if the crystals are placed directly on the tongue, it produces a cooling sensation, but no unpleasant flavors. The cooling feeling is not noticeable when added to foods, however, making erythritol an excellent sugar substitute. It is the one to use, although it can be fortified, to make it sweeter.

Monk fruit extract is another super-sweet set of non-caloric compounds, with a long history of use in China. I have a stock of monk fruit sweetener formulated in erythritol, which is exactly as sweet as sugar, is crystalline like sugar, and is not distinguishable from sugar at any useful concentration. The only reservation I have about monk fruit is that it is so similar to sugar, it even tickles the insulin response. It is a major theme of this book that this is not a great thing, and because of that, I avoid consuming it regularly. On the other hand, I don't use any sweeteners regularly, anymore. But in an occasional desert, I have no reservations about monk fruit sweetener.

Regularity and Fiber

Fiber is a carbohydrate. However, it is not metabolized like other carbohydrates, leading to the term, *net carbohydrates*, or net carbs. Total carbs, minus fiber, equals net carbs. Net carbs come from sugars and starch, and are what we classically consider carbs. They are quickly digested, and elevate blood glucose levels. Fiber, on the other hand, is associated with *smooth moves*, in the sense of the absence of constipation. Fiber is in fruits, vegetables, and even whole grains. So long as fruits and grains were eaten whole, metabolic syndrome was a non-issue. It was the advent of refined carbs and sugars that tipped the scales in the wrong direction. So is fiber a good thing, no questions asked? Alas, opinions on fiber are varied in the ketogenic dieting literature.

First, a distinction must be made between two kinds of fiber. Insoluble fiber, or cellulose, is inert in the digestive tract. It is composed of glucose units, joined in a way that mammals cannot digest. Herbivores have bacteria in their guts that do the digesting, and produce all sorts of nutrients in the process. To them, a handful of grass must look like a plate of spaghetti. But to us, it is inert. Sawdust is essentially the same thing. I have a stock of oat fiber, which tastes exactly like sawdust, and which I will probably never use up.

A second type of fiber is soluble fiber. It is a highly hydrated, complex molecule. It is the fiber found in psyllium husk, the active ingredient in Metamucil, and other fiber supplements. When soluble and insoluble fiber occur together, the insoluble fiber forms a solid support for the soluble fiber to attach to, and form a gooey substance with the consistency of, well, the topic of this section. So it would seem, based on the above, that the more fiber one can eat, the better, right?

The reason opinions are divided is because soluble fiber is not entirely inert in the gut. Some of it is fermented by gut bacteria, and the resulting metabolites can be used by the intestines to synthesize glucose. The process is called intestinal gluconeogenesis. For reasons I don't presently understand, this is known to produce a *decrease* in actual blood glucose. That fact is cited by some, to prove it is good. We've already discussed how short-term increases or decreases in blood glucose should not be yardsticks by which we judge a nutritional question. It should be overall health. Too much soluble fiber can produce enough glucose to put a person out of ketosis. As a result of that observation, many ketogenic dieters count fiber together with their total carbohydrates, as they strive to limit all sources of carb. But in fairness, those people are setting a ketone number as the surrogate marker of health, and that is not inherently different from using a blood glucose number. So where does the truth lie?

On one hand, starches and sugars are completely absorbed by the digestive system, and increase glucose load far more than a similar amount of fiber. Only a small fraction of the mass of soluble fiber can ever be converted to glucose. And someone who avoided too much fiber might avoid avocados, a delicious and healthy fruit that goes so well with bacon and eggs, because it has a significant amount of soluble fiber. If food science was truly advanced, we might have access to a conversion factor, where a certain amount of soluble fiber will, through fermentation and intestinal gluconeogenesis, produce something like 1% of its mass in glucose. Or it could be 5%. I have not found data on the question. But even if I did, or made a guess, there is still the problem that nutrition labels do not separate out soluble versus insoluble fiber. So different foods will produce different outcomes. And a question I will return to at the end is, *Is it ketosis* per se *that I am trying to achieve, or are ketones merely a marker of an insulin response at rest*? If soluble fiber will on occasion compromise ketosis, does it also result in elevated insulin? Not having answers to these questions, I don't worry too much whether an occasional meal has too much soluble fiber. Variety of food is an important health factor, for the simple reason that our biochemical needs are not fully defined. The various micronutrients in various foods all matter, in the long run.

As I made my transition to ketosis, I quickly learned I could no longer eat ordinary oatmeal in the morning, due to its high carb content. I've always had a love-hate relationship with oatmeal. I used to eat it to keep myself regular, and it did that job very well. And I ate it unsweetened, only adding a few frozen blueberries for some flavor, and antioxidants. But I've always hated the taste and texture of oatmeal. It was simply the best thing I could find, to keep me regular. As I gave up oatmeal, and before I learned the nuances of low carb dieting, I developed a problem with constipation. Eating a lot of salad will solve the problem, but it makes the stuff in back push and shove extra hard, trying to be first to get out. That can be uncomfortable. The next prescription is to add magnesium oxide as a supplement. That form of magnesium is insoluble, so very little is absorbed, and is not an effective dietary supplement. But it is a potent laxative. Too potent, to the point where accidents are possible. That's not fun when my daily walk is an hour through residential neighborhoods. My biggest fear is that I'd have to pound on a stranger's door, twisting and grimacing in pain, and begging to use the facilities.

Heavy consumption of difficult to digest snacks, such as nuts and cheese, may constipate, but these foods are staples of the ketogenic diet. At some point, most ketogenic dieters will attempt to achieve regularity with fiber supplements, which usually consist of psyllium husk (soluble fiber). This produces a gel-like consistency, and results in smoother movements. But without accompanying insoluble fiber, psyllium husk is only modestly effective at lower amounts.

What works best for me are probiotics, otherwise known as bacterial supplements. Yes, our guts are full of all sorts of bacteria. A newborn baby drinking breast milk quickly has its gut colonized by lactobacilli, germs that specialize in fermenting the lactose in milk that is not absorbed in the upper part of the digestive system. And as any parent knows, newborns fed breast milk do not suffer from constipation. Constipation only happens if fed formula fortified with free iron, or once they are consuming mostly solid food. In either case, the bacterial composition of the gut changes in an unfavorable way.

In the same way, lactobacilli can keep adult colons working smoothly. There are several ways to get lactobacilli. One is to take pills containing them. Another is to eat live cultures of lactobacilli, otherwise known as yogurt. At our house, we make our own yogurt, using a $50 yogurt maker (opt for one with a glass jar, rather than plastic). We use whole milk and half and half, in whatever proportion is available, but the more half and half, the creamier and tastier the final product. Advice I've seen is to start with your favorite commercial plain yogurt, and use it as a starter culture. We like FAGE best. Ours usually comes out as rich as the best Greek yogurts on the market, and not as sour. Like so many others who make their own yogurt, we've come to prefer it over the commercial varieties, and even with our pricey ingredients, ours costs much less than store bought yogurt. We don't sweeten, as I believe in losing the sweet taste, but I would not object to occasionally adding some erythritol, if weaning off the sweet tooth has to be done more gradually.

But I do not believe yogurt is okay, in unlimited amounts. Moderation still holds as the rule. Traces of lactose remain in yogurt, and it is not very sweet, so its presence is not easily detected. Too much yogurt, and my weight will climb. Whenever a change in diet results in weight gain, I experiment with reversing it. If the weight comes off, then that change was a factor in the weight gain.

Summary: Some fraction of soluble fiber can be converted to glucose, and a lot of soluble fiber can put one out of ketosis. Some count fiber as a carb for this reason, even though little is absorbed as glucose. I don't worry if an occasional meal will put me out of ketosis, if I'm getting a good variety of micronutrients from my food. Too many nuts can constipate, and for some, too much cheese. Yogurt or lactobacilli pills (probiotics) can keep things moving smoothly.

Fine Tuning the Diet

Food is more than mere nourishment. It is a source of comfort, that draws on childhood memories of contentment. So I don't believe anyone can simply throw away all the foods they've ever known, memorize some fifty new recipes from cookbooks, and be truly satisfied with their new diet. Such a radical change would leave you psychologically stressed, while you're trying to beat diabetes, which is worsened by stress. The trick has to be finding ways to eliminate the carbs from favorite recipes, and yet retain that sense of familiarity that characterizes our favorites. Only then can a person really be satisfied. As I learned I had to increase my fat intake, I had to adapt favorite recipes to my new regimen. If I made burritos for the family, they got a conventional burrito, in a regular

120

tortilla. But a single small flour tortilla has 20 grams of carbohydrates, which is 100% of my daily limit. And I have to factor in that every food has traces of carb, so every gram or two counts. 20 grams of carb in one tortilla is out of the question. What to do? I tried low-carb tortillas, containing only 6 grams of carb (made with oat fiber), and they taste like cardboard. I did not long flirt with that solution. Eventually, I decided to simply try going without any tortilla, or made one by frying a layer of shredded cheese.

After my glucose came down into the range of 150 mg/dl (about three weeks in), I hit my first roadblock. I could exercise, and get my glucose to come down into the 130s, but it would quickly shoot back up into the 150 range. A little reading, and I found the explanation. Too much protein is equivalent to glucose. The ketogenic dieting guides are very clear about this point. When the liver converts excess protein to glucose, the body does not enter ketosis, even if the appearance of that new glucose is slow, and does not cause a spike. I had to adjust my diet, and cut back on protein. Gone were the days of a big steak, or even steak and salad without any potatoes. I also had to add calories from fat.

My original objective was not to enter into ketosis, but simply to reduce my blood glucose. I had not yet formulated a big picture vision of overall health. In spite of good measurements throughout the day, including after dinner, I would again top 150 mg/dl the following morning. It was now approaching a month since I started, and I never wanted to see 150 mg/dl on the glucose meter again. By this time, I had read books on ketogenic dieting, and learned that sustainable nutritional ketosis is not possible while blood glucose is above 150 mg/dl. Taking a tip from Jimmy Moore's book, *Keto Clarity*, and not having thought through the implications, I agreed to a prescription for metformin, at a dose of 500 mg.

I took my first dose of metformin before bed time, contrary to the regular, morning dosing schedule. I thought I had a good reason for this, as I was still discovering the particulars of the morning glucose spike. I decided that the only way my fasting glucose could be higher in the morning than it was the previous evening, several hours after my last meal, was if my liver spent the night converting excess protein into new glucose. The process is called *gluconeogenesis*. Both of limiting my meat intake, and taking metformin, were aimed at combating this. The liver will not work as hard to make glucose, if protein is not in excess, and metformin activates the cell starvation response, that stimulates glucose uptake and inhibits gluconeogenesis.

The results were immediate. Over the next week, my highest morning glucose reading was 133 mg/dl. But was it metformin, or cutting my protein, that was responsible? If my intention was to conduct scientific experiments on myself, I would only change one variable at a time. But my intention was to cut my glucose first, and only later worry about how I got there.

One evening, about a week later, I forgot to take metformin. I only realized it when I was already in bed, and almost asleep. I thought for a moment, and decided not to take it, so I could see the effect the following morning. In the morning, I measured 131 mg/dl. It was within the range of measurements over the previous week. I deliberately left out metformin again that night, and the next morning, measured 134 mg/dl. Broadly speaking, that was the same number. I took metformin again that night, and followed with a measurement of 129 mg/dl the following morning. I tried a week with metformin, a week without, and quickly learned it made no difference, on average. That left the conscious reduction in meat as the variable responsible for getting my glucose below 150 mg/dl.

What I learned subsequently is that metformin wears off after about six hours. Okay, so I was still getting its action for much of the night, but come morning, the effect was gone. And my problem was not a middle of the night problem, but a morning problem. I subsequently tried metformin during the day, and found any effect to be slight, at best. So slight, I can't say with confidence that it was even real. With that, I dropped it, and never finished my second 30 day prescription. I was doing better with diet than with drugs.

It was also at this time that I became aware of the inaccuracy of glucose meters. When a morning measurement came in near my long-term average, I did not question it. But when a measurement was aberrant, I measured it again, with a second strip, or a different glucose meter. Only by becoming aware of the lack of reproducibility, and taking enough measurements to understand what was real, could I be sure when my numbers truly spiked in the morning. And if I had eaten normally, and everything else was in order, I learned that an unusually high morning glucose spike meant

I was probably getting sick. Within a few days, I would develop cold symptoms. And a day or two later, my glucose would decline again.

My first sub-100 morning measurement came about two and a half months in. And it was not the glorious moment I had imagined it might be. The truth is, it was over the Christmas-New Year holiday period, and I awoke a little bit under the weather from a few drinks the previous night. I measured my morning glucose at 93 mg/dl. Not trusting the measurement, I repeated it, and it came back at 100 mg/dl. Twice in a tight range, and I start to believe the measurement. Time to celebrate? Not quite. The truth is, my liver had been busy that night, metabolizing alcohol, and turning it into fat. Being preoccupied, its capacity to create new glucose was impaired. Add to that the insulin sensitizing effect of alcohol, and the morning spike would be blunted. A telling fact is that I did not measure another sub-100 morning reading for several weeks (although I was usually measuring below 100 in the afternoon). Over time, my experiences with alcohol are consistent. Drinking a little too much will reduce my glucose reading the following morning. Time to order cases and cases of my favorite wines? Well, no. Alcohol consumption builds fat, which over the long term, works against controlling blood glucose. Accordingly, daily alcohol consumption to reduce blood glucose is counterproductive over the long run. This is another example of not putting the short-term surrogate marker (morning blood glucose) ahead of actual health. Drinking will improve the surrogate right away, but can harm overall health, and worsen the surrogate over time.

Initially, I wanted to reduce my glucose so desperately that I was willing to forego any indulgence. But over time, as I began to feel like I was succeeding, I started to want some sense of normalcy back in my life. And over holiday periods, many of us end up drinking regularly, as well as eating a less controlled diet. At my house, we have adapted desserts with non-glycemic sweeteners that do not affect ketosis, but which by their sweetness, may stimulate insulin secretion. One might find a blood glucose reduction after such a dessert, but I have suspicions that this may not be a good thing, over the long term. The insulin signal is still the bad guy in this whole story, so the objective continues to be to use it as little as possible. On one hand, there is no bolus of glucose for the body to work with.

On the other, the secretion of insulin stimulates the fat cells first, as they are last to become insulin resistant. They will take up what glucose there is in circulation, and use it to generate a pool of glycerol. Then, the fat in the diet can be stabilized in those fat cells, and weight gain occurs. Desserts (non-glycemic, of course) on special occasions are a part of our lives, so we allow them. But we won't make them routine.

Special occasions also involve more alcohol consumption than normal, so it is difficult to point to a single factor, but I reliably come out of those times heavier, often with higher morning glucose measurements. Fortunately, I can reverse this over the next couple of weeks, by cutting out desserts and at least on weekdays, alcohol, and maintaining a regular exercise regimen.

By about three months after starting, my morning blood glucose was very stable, other than at the start of a viral infection. I would reliably measure between 90 mg/dl and about 115 mg/dl. I would measure at the low or high end of the range for a week or two at a time, and then see a change. As a rule, my afternoon numbers were below 100 mg/dl. I still wanted to reduce my morning numbers to reliably below 100 mg/dl, but I suspected it would not come quickly. It's possible I was in this range, just over 100 mg/dl, for many years, and it could be my body's interpretation of normal. Later, I concluded that my stress responses are exaggerated, and chronically elevated cortisol keeps my glucose slightly elevated. But it is close enough to normal that it is no longer a cause for concern, especially when it's only for a few hours each morning. Healthy carb-eaters spike a lot higher than that after a meal. Accordingly, I tweaked my primary goal. I continue to monitor my glucose, but usually only in the morning, with sporadic measurements at other times, especially if I feel like it might be off in some way. But I made it my primary goal to be in nutritional ketosis most of the time. That's an excellent indication that my insulin response is not being used.

Summary: As rapidly as weight came off, it ended as abruptly when I reached my historic waist size. Getting below 150 mg/dl blood glucose required limiting protein intake. After a short trial with metformin, I decided it was not doing anything, and stopped taking it. Alcohol will reduce my morning blood glucose, but my weight will climb when I drink more regularly. After a while, my baseline morning glucose will increase. Stopping alcohol reverses both in short order.

Changing Shopping Habits

Suddenly, the grocery store became a much smaller place. On a high fat low carb diet, you find yourself avoiding entire blocks of aisles in grocery stores. I have come to appreciate that they bundle all the processed foods together, and all the carb-intensive junk food together, to make avoiding it simple. My wife or I will occasionally stop in the junk food section to pick up some pork rinds, and in the drinks section to pick up some seltzer, but I don't remember the last time we bought food in a box. What now comes home from the grocery store would generally be familiar to my ancestors from two hundred years ago.

I sometimes shop at Costco, and before long noticed I was avoiding every single one of those free sample booths they set up at the ends of the aisles. It's nearly certain that every last one is sweetened, or carb-rich. At first, I shuddered as I passed, sometimes muttering under my breath, "If you only knew what that does to you..." Then, one day, I had a thought. It has to be costly to pay someone to stand there and push those products. And grocery stores operate on famously thin margins. So if the return justifies the cost, carb-rich products must be especially profitable. Perhaps it is no accident that every last one of those products is carb-rich.

In general, the more processed a food is, the more carbs it has. Replacing fat or protein with carb is a sure way to make foods cheaper to produce, more stable in transit, and therefore more profitable. Perhaps this helps explain the resistance of the broader system to call out carbs for what they are. There is too much money in them.

A trip to the grocery store starts in produce, where we typically like to stock a variety of vegetables. Many meals consist of a meat, a fatty sauce, and some steamed broccoli, green beans, or other green vegetables. The children have learned to love Brussels sprouts, as a curiosity. Of course, it doesn't hurt that after boiling, we quickly fry them up on bacon fat, and serve them with crumbled bacon. We buy carrots for the children, and I usually limit myself to only a few. But I won't avoid them altogether, because of the retinoid compounds they contain in abundance. Squashes are surprisingly low in carbs, as long as they are eaten in reasonable amounts. A whole zucchini only has six grams of net carbs, for instance. Tomatoes are reasonably low in carb, with about five grams per tomato. Cabbage is fine. Cucumbers are good, as are snow peas (in the whole pod). Turnips, rutabagas, and parsnips are good for soups, or even to eat steamed, in place of potatoes. The only concern is that while one zucchini is okay by itself, three would approach my daily limit. The same tends to be true of many other vegetables, so three servings of different vegetables could approach my limit. A zucchini, a tomato, and a cup of snow peas, for instance, might be too much, when accounting for other sources of glucose over the course of the day. But even then, I will do it on occasion, if the nutritional quality of the food in question justifies it. Leafy vegetables are reliably low in carbs, so salads made with various types of lettuce, assorted greens, and spinach, make for good side dishes.

Next stop, fruits. Most fruits are not compatible with low carb diets, even if most are fine for healthy people. The sugar they contain is offset by the fiber, and so its absorption is slowed sufficiently that the liver can burn the fructose. But many people are surprised to learn how nutrient-poor fruits are. Grapes are mostly natural bags of sugar-water, for instance. We buy bananas for the rest of the family, but for me, a single one is above my daily carb limit. Ditto for apples. Interestingly, a single banana does not seem to raise my blood glucose at all (I've tested it). Strawberries are low in sugar, again subject to eating a modest serving. Small amounts of wild blueberries are fine, and rich in antioxidants. The cultivated ones may have too much sugar.

Next stop, the bulk bins. Almond flour is a staple at my house, as is coconut flour. Both are low in carb, and can be used to simulate many flour based foods. Next, oils. Coconut oil is a favorite, and we buy the refined variety, rather than virgin, or the meaningless marketing term they hope will evoke olive oil, *extra virgin*. Coconut oil is refined with steam, a clean process, and it removes any coconut flavors from the final product. It's only a matter of preference, and flexibility, since coconut flavors are fine with some foods, but don't agree with many others. Some people still eschew coconut oil, because it is a saturated fat. But coconut oil consists of medium chain triglycerides, which means the saturated fat molecules are of a medium length. The consequence is that they are too short to be stored in fat cells, and are burned directly, either as straight fats, or as ketones, converted by the liver. And when used for frying, coconut oil is highly resistant to oxidation, making it perhaps the healthiest oil for that purpose.

We always try to keep some lard at home. Stores almost seem embarrassed to sell lard, and at least in California, often only call it *manteca*, its Spanish name. A pot of soup that tastes a little thin can be transformed into a deliciously rich dish with a cup of lard thrown in. We also keep olive oil, and avocado oil, and often blend it with coconut oil for frying, especially for vegetables. Olive and avocado oils have similar fat profiles, but avocado oil is comparatively tasteless, for when that makes a difference. Butter is technically a dairy item, but we also go through a lot, whether for frying certain things, or melting it on vegetables. Under no circumstances would we buy canola oil, soybean oil, or any other vegetable oil. They are all very rich in inflammatory omega-6 oils, and have no history in the human diet. To the extent that the first humans ever ate legumes or seeds containing those oils, it was never more than a tiny fraction of the amount it takes to make even a few drops of oil. Today's hyper-production of those oils on an industrial scale ensures they are cheap, available, and endorsed, but this is at odds with their health effects. I retired an existing flask of canola oil, and now use it as paint thinner. It works very well for that purpose, and is far less noxious than turpentine or mineral spirits.

After that, it's on to the meats. To the surprise of some who have not thought through the whole concept, going high fat, low carb has saved us money on meat. First stop, ground beef. Forget about the lean stuff. Go for the cheaper, fatty ground beef. Next, some pork shoulder meat, for marinating and making shish kebabs. Ignore any pricey, lean meats. People often talk of grass-fed beef, rather than grain-fed, as a way of producing better fat profiles in the meat. I don't often see that option in grocery stores, but if you do, and can trust it's the truth, go for it. It's the same question for anything labeled *organic*. Sure, we'd like our food free of pesticides, but how confident are you about how tightly it's enforced? Occasionally, a lean cut of meat may be the only choice for certain dishes, in which case you'll need to make a fatty sauce to accompany it. And that takes us to the next stop: Dairy.

If eggs can be considered dairy, then here's the place. Stock a lot of eggs, and eat them often, including the yolks. Next, heavy cream. The higher the fat content, the better. It will be used in everything from coffee to sauce with meat, to the occasional dessert. After that, get a big tub of cream cheese, and another of sour cream. You never want to be caught without these two staples. And don't forget a lot of butter.

Then there's cheese. Full fat shredded mozzarella is an essential staple. Some shredded parmesan/romano is another good addition, to give those sauces a little more flavor. Also get some shredded cheddar-jack, for any kind of Mexican recipe. It is also useful to have a block of your favorite hard cheese, for when dinner was not fatty enough, and you're left hungry. Two slices of cheese can form a sandwich, containing thick slabs of butter, and a small slice of salami, or other flavorful meat.

At some point, we pass the baking aisle. Cocoa powder is a major item on our list, as is some powdered milk. These, plus some cocoa butter (you have to get that online, in my experience) and coconut oil will make a fabulous and healthy chocolate.

Finally, there's milk. Adults should not drink milk straight, because of the lactose content. But children will protest if their parents try to deny them. I make sure to avoid reduced fat milks. Those that buy skim milk subsidize those of us who buy the fat taken from those milks, and put it into butter, cream, and derived products. Yet another example where the system works in our favor.

By avoiding the aisles where they keep cereals, bread, juices, bottled drinks and boxed dinners, shopping trips are much quicker, cheaper, and healthier.

Summary: Shopping is easier when avoiding carbs. Junk food, processed food aisles are simply passed by. We buy a lot of vegetables, fatty meats, and full fat dairy products. Coconut and almond flour for certain recipes. We use olive oil, butter and coconut oil for cooking.

Chapter 7: Stressing Over the Details

Kindness and a generous spirit go a long way. And a sense of humor. It's like medicine - very healing. ~ Max Irons

The Morning Glucose Spike

I've now read the accounts of other post-diabetics. I've seen it called *remission*, but I really hate that name. I was a cancer researcher, after all, where remission is usually considered temporary. Back to post-diabetes: Every case I'm familiar with recounts the same thing. The morning blood glucose number is the high for the day. It is a spike, and nothing related to diet or exercise seems to solve it. Learning what was behind it was the last piece of the puzzle, as I put this book together.

When I first noticed the pattern of blood glucose spiking in the morning, I decided to track it over the course of a morning. On waking, I measured 97 mg/dl. So far, so good. I passed on my morning coffee, drinking only water. I even deferred my supplements, so literally all I had that morning was plain water. Two hours later, I measured again, and read 107 mg/dl. Another two hours, and I measured 112 mg/dl. On one hand, these measurements are within the margin of error considered acceptable for glucose meters, which is disconcerting. But the trend caught my eye, so I repeated it on several additional days. Each time, the trend was intact. My glucose would rise over the course of the morning, until I ate. Then, it would decline. Eventually, I persuaded myself that the trend was real. Is this normal? The glucose comes from the liver, and producing some is probably part of the daily cycle of waking and getting ready to function for the day. You might even predict that everyone's glucose rises as they get up in the morning. Fortunately, I was able to test this assumption, because I have a willing guinea pig, living with me.

I decided to measure my wife's glucose. When I began our collective journey away from carbs, I measured her glucose one morning, and it was 92 mg/dl. She's never had any blood glucose issues. By this time, many months later, she had adjusted to a diet closer to HFLC, although she had not yet adopted a strict adherence to it. I explained my theory about morning glucose spikes, and she agreed to several measurements one morning. So I measured her glucose at waking, and it was 73 mg/dl. She got her glucose a whole lot lower, with a lot less rigor to her diet, by simply approximating what I was doing. My next question was what would happen over the course of the next few hours, before she ate anything. She agreed, and I measured her glucose again 45 minutes later. It came back at 74 mg/dl. An identical reading. The same morning, I measured my glucose at waking, and it was 96 mg/dl. After measuring hers for the second time, I also measured mine again: 107 mg/dl. The trend was intact. Mine rises, while hers does not. I suspect we're both mobilizing our glucose reserves on waking, but her system was in equilibrium, where I still had an underlying issue.

What is it that makes that morning number spike? A clue came when I switched to daylight savings time, the first year I was low-carb. This was in the spring, when we wake an hour earlier, and it takes a few days to adapt to the new schedule. The previous week, I was recording morning numbers in the 110 mg/dl range, but the first week of daylight savings time, I measured below 100 mg/dl. But the end of the week came around, and suddenly I reverted to the range I had previously had, in the 100-110 mg/dl range. What happened? The answer, it seems, is that my body adjusted to waking up early, and timed the glucose spike to arrive earlier than it previously had. After this experience, I made a point of taking a measurement any time I had to wake early, and the trend was beyond dispute. As little as forty minutes early and my number was below what I measured the day before or after. It really appears to be a short-lived spike in blood glucose, at exactly the time I normally wake up.

The process of waking up is a lot more complex than opening your eyes, and forcing yourself out of bed. The unconscious parts of the brain know roughly when it is time to wake up, and orchestrate a set of responses to ensure that extra glucose is available in the morning. It's part of what is known as the circadian clock, and is perfectly normal. Want to know what your blood glucose is all night? Wake an hour early, and measure it then.

I had all but given up trying to neutralize the morning glucose spike with diet and exercise. It was closing in on two years, and it would still come and go, unpredictably. Some weeks I was below 100 mg/dl, some weeks above. It was a reminder of diabetes, so I really wanted to make it go away, but I could not find a reliable way to keep it down. At first, I tried to link it to cycles of weight gain or loss, and that may yet play a role, but the correlation was weak. I was flummoxed. Even if the size of the spike was not alarming, it was a puzzle. Had I damaged my endocrine system in some permanent way? Was there something else I was not aware of?

At one point, I researched what it was that made glucose spike in the morning, and quickly came across the stress hormone, cortisol. It also spikes in the morning, and raises blood glucose. For a long time, I did not give this a second thought. Stress is a neurological thing, and I like biochemical pathways, where you can draw a clean diagram with arrows connecting everything. Eventually, I came across stress in different contexts, including as a contributing cause of diabetes, and decided I had to look into it a little deeper. That topic is next.

Summary: The morning glucose spike is caused by cortisol, the stress hormone. It is also a contributing cause of diabetes.

Stress and the HPA Axis

Chronic stress is a contributing cause of heart disease. This is not a controversial idea. But does it play a role in diabetes? Like the medical system itself, I was initially reluctant to embrace the idea of stress in disease. It's too subjective, and if you asked me to rank my stress level, I would see it as an invitation to engage in self-pity, or to make excuses. *It's not my fault I have diabetes, it's the stress I was under.* So it was with some reluctance that I came to accept that stress is a relevant thing.

What is stress? I think of it as heightened anxiety and tension, on a constant basis, but without a good resolution in sight. We all face tension and anxiety, but if we have reasons for optimism, those are usually manageable. Anyone who has to meet a tight deadline experiences stress, but once the deadline is met, the stress is relieved. You can even emerge stronger for it, meaning it's probably a healthy manifestation of stress. It's when you're trapped in a bad situation, with no hope of a good outcome, that stress becomes pathological. How?

Let's introduce the HPA Axis. The term evokes an *axis* as an alliance of enemies, and we're only aware of the HPA Axis when it goes bad. HPA stands for hypothalamus, pituitary, and adrenal cortex.

The hypothalamus is the principal interface between the nervous system and the endocrine system. If there's a place where something goes wrong in one, and affects the other, it is going to be here. One of the functions of the hypothalamus is to respond to neurological stress, and produce corticotropin releasing hormone (CRH). CRH travels only a short distance, to the pituitary gland, where it triggers the release of corticotropin. Corticotropin travels through the blood, to the cortex of the adrenal glands, where it stimulates release of the principal stress hormone, cortisol. Among the functions of cortisol is to raise blood glucose levels, to help combat the source of the stress. It also raises blood pressure, and suppresses the immune system, yet causes inflammation. But we also use cortisol cream, called hydrocortisone, to suppress inflammation on the skin. Clearly, the system is much more complex than is presently understood.

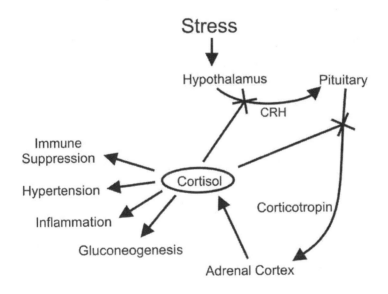

When the HPA Axis is functioning properly, cortisol inhibits the release of more CRH and corticotropin. It's a typical feedback inhibition loop, and it limits the duration of the stress response. If there is to be more firing of the HPA Axis, it has to come from more stress from the nervous system, triggering the hypothalamus to produce more CRH. The system works as a way of translating stress at the neurological level into physiological responses, which are referred to as *downstream effects*. The HPA Axis works together with the autonomic nervous system, and in the short term, prepares the body to combat whatever stressful situation it is faced with.

But for those under chronic stress, the negative feedback loop weakens, as gene expression patterns are changed by epigenetic mechanisms (which are more stable over time). There is debate about whether these changes may be determined early in development, as a response to childhood stress, or in adulthood. There are even suggestions that repeated concussions may contribute (such as would be experienced by hockey goalies getting hit in the head with hockey pucks?). There is little debate that a substantial fraction of those with signs of chronic stress, addiction, and many behavioral disorders, have impaired HPA Axis function. And those people have elevated risks of heart disease, diabetes, and probably other diseases. If the effects of diabetes were not so obviously implicated in heart disease risk, one might even speculate that heart disease and diabetes are two independent manifestations of HPA Axis dysfunction.

Those with HPA Axis dysfunction are going to have stronger, and longer, cortisol -driven stress responses than those for whom the negative feedback is working properly. Their blood glucose will remain elevated longer, resulting in more insulin secretion, and more insulin resistance. It should be obvious by now that this represents a possible path to diabetes. All that is missing is the fuel to launch that rocket: Carbs.

I am aware that I have an elevated and prolonged stress response, and probably always did. Furthermore, some years before I learned I was diabetic, I went through a stressful period in my life. I put on weight, and in retrospect, it's easy to point to that time and say that's when I became diabetic. So how big a role did stress play in my developing diabetes? I was carb-fed at the time. I even put sugar in my coffee, back then. So how does one separate the various factors? You can't, with any scientific rigor. I believe stress played a role, but I don't believe I could have progressed to full diabetes without the carbs. On what do I base that?

The stressful period ended a good five years before I learned I was diabetic. I was probably diabetic for much of those five years without knowing it. My stress levels rose and fell over that time, but the diabetes remained. Then, when I changed my diet, I cut my blood glucose by half in the first three weeks. My stress had not vanished, and it continued to come and go, afterwards.

Can elimination of stress reverse full-blown diabetes? Based on my history, I'm guessing not. Further, I think it's impossible to eliminate stress altogether. I'm not about to become a monk and move to the Himalayas, but even if I did, something there would eventually stress me out. Secondly, I think stress is a trigger that accelerates the escalation of the insulin resistance feedback loop, but not the principal fuel. But I'm not dogmatic. I broke the feedback loop with my diet, but if someone wants to try breaking it with meditation, and other stress relief measures, I won't dissuade the initiative. Use your glucose meter to judge the merit of any idea you want to try. Does it lead to being able to cut down or discontinue diabetes medications in a short time? Don't waste too much time if the improvement is not rapid.

In only a few minutes of searching, I found three drugs that block the CRH receptor on the pituitary gland, and thus promise to blunt the stress response. Antalarmin is from Pfizer, Pexacerfont from Bristol Myers Squibb, and Verucerfont from GlaxoSmithKline. According to Wikipedia, *initial results have been disappointing, when testing these drugs on anxiety related disorders.* Now, go back and read this section again if you need to, and especially if you work for any of the above drug companies. Anxiety comes first, cortisol comes second. Cortisol transmits the signal from the nervous system to the rest of the body. So testing these drugs for anxiety and related disorders is like building a dam on a river, and later expressing disappointment that it has not improved flooding *upstream*. The potential for these drugs is in combating diabetes and heart disease. If the right people were targeted, they could conceivably meet the ever-elusive standard of all-cause mortality benefit, and might be able to report absolute risk, rather than relative risk, without being sneered at by those in the know.

Trials to validate these drugs would be expensive, even if they showed an obvious benefit. If the patents do not extend far enough into the future, there is no chance to recoup the investment. That's too bad, because I'd find it very amusing to see how quickly the medical bandwagon could change its principal focus. Suddenly, the *saturated fat-cholesterol-statin* story would morph into a, *forget fat, it's stress* story. The major news networks would be full of reports on the dangers posed by stress, complete with expert interviews every day, and you could not tune out the subject without unplugging from the world. The drugs would make their grand entry just as the coverage reached its crescendo, and would quickly become the world's best-selling drugs, advertised non-stop on the same networks that helped hype the problem. And in spite of myself, I think that could actually be a good development. In spite of their probably high costs, such drugs could save money for the system, overall.

Summary: Stress plays a role in the development of both diabetes and heart disease. The HPA axis mediates, and limits, the stress response, but chronic stress weakens the negative feedback. Stress responses are stronger, and longer lived. My stress level makes the difference between normal morning glucose and post-diabetic morning glucose numbers.

Alcohol/Fructohol

It bears repeating that overall health is not an isolated blood glucose number, or even that plus several other measurements, thrown in. Properly chosen surrogate markers correlate well with overall health, but treatments that target surrogate markers without fixing the underlying disease may not improve overall health. The example of alcohol is highly pertinent to this topic, because drinking can result in a lower morning blood glucose value. If the surrogate marker of morning blood glucose was the only relevant consideration, we would say, "Aha! I'll just get drunk every night, and my problem will be solved." And this would be dead wrong, because the surrogate is only one measure which, if altered in isolation, does not improve overall health.

On one doctors' visit, she insisted on a follow-up blood test, as it was about seven months since my last one. I was still confident that everything was moving in the right direction, when she called with my results. She acknowledged that I did a good job getting my HbA1C down to 6%, from a previous 11% (and probably about 13% before being measured), but there was a disapproving tone in her voice. My HDL went up from the mid forties to the mid sixties, which is officially considered protective against heart disease, but

135

neither did that earn me any praise. She then pointed out that my LDL was elevated, which I expected, and did not fear. But my triglycerides and VLDL were also significantly elevated. This made no sense at all. As my mind was running through why this could be, she added that this was, "probably from your ketogenic diet," and reiterated the standard dietary advice that had failed me for so long. If she could have handed me another copy of the food pyramid flier through the phone, I expect she would have.

The news made me feel vulnerable, and tied my tongue. I should have corrected her error in attributing high triglycerides to a ketogenic diet, but could not muster the wit at that time. I expected my HDL to be up, and it was. But I expected my triglycerides to be down, and they were up. *Where were they coming from?* Extensive reading after the fact confirmed that blood triglycerides come from carbohydrates in the diet, and not from fats. There are no known conditions that cause the reverse. My doctor clearly did not understand the relationship between diet and lipid profiles, or the ketogenic diet. But how could I refute her, when I had this strange result?

Extensive reading failed to turn up an answer. The quickly growing minority of doctors who support the ketogenic lifestyle measure triglycerides to determine whether the patient is a *carbaholic*. Yet at the time, I was measuring robust levels of ketones in my urine; a virtual guarantee that I was effectively abstaining from carbs, I thought. Confused, I slowly developed doubts about what I was trying to accomplish. With a new level of uncertainty, I strayed from the high fat element of the diet over that summer, and incorporated more vegetables. It was not because I felt this would fix my problem. I did not know how to fix the problem. It was because my doubts led me to compromise on my diet, an echo of those years of indoctrination that fats were bad. By the fall (twelve months into my journey), I had put on about five pounds, and over the winter, another ten. In retrospect, this is to be expected, once the high fat element of the diet is compromised. I grew hungry more often, and took to peanuts as a snack. A handful of peanuts is okay. But a bowl full starts to raise carb levels to where the insulin response takes notice.

My urine ketone readings faded by about nine months, and were soon undetectable. *Surely I had not reverted that badly.* My blood glucose crept up also, where the average morning reading used to be below 110 mg/dl, it was now about 120 mg/dl. Was the diet failing me, or was I failing the diet? My doctor was no help, and I couldn't find any answers on my own. *If I can't find answers to these questions*, I thought, *who can?* In retrospect, the lack of a good support system at that moment was particularly discouraging. I had no idea what to do. Should I weigh my glucose reduction and elevated HDL (good) against my triglycerides and VLDL (bad)? I never felt like giving up, but I became unnerved, and softened my high fat diet as a result.

In that time frame, I came across an article written by cardiac surgeon and University of Washington professor Donald W. Miller, who has embraced high fat diets. I reached out to him by email, and besides discussing an aspect of his article, I mentioned my situation. His response was a thing of beauty: "The way I deal with blood tests ordered by guideline-following physicians is to simply not do them. I haven't had mine done in decades. I'm 76, and I feel great. Why go through the trauma of the test, when the advice that follows will be wrong, anyway?" He has made similar comments publicly, and has a popular video on Youtube (code vRe9z32NZHY), titled *Enjoy Eating Saturated Fats: They're Good for You*. His advice raised my spirits immediately, and I have taken it to heart. Whatever the results that came back, my approach would only be to redouble my efforts to rid myself of carbs. But I still lacked an explanation for my unusual lab profile, and weight gain.

A turning point came when the season of Lent arrived. I customarily give up alcohol during Lent, and did so again this year. Over those six weeks, I dropped all the weight I had put on over the previous year, and my average morning glucose dropped down into the low 100s. It was dramatic, and served as a stark reminder that alcohol limits the success of the ketogenic diet. I then reviewed everything I had experienced to that point.

Shortly after my return home on discovering I was diabetic, I quit alcohol cold turkey, for about a month. My first blood test was well into this *dry* window. But after I made so much progress in such a short time, I gradually began to increase my frequency and quantity of alcohol, eventually approximating what I used to do before learning of my diabetes. I would rarely, if ever, drink alcohol before about eight pm. After eight, depending on the mood, I might have a Manhattan, made with about 2-3 ounces of whiskey, or a Martini with a similar amount of vodka. If wine, it would be about two glasses. I turn in for the night between ten and eleven pm. But at certain times, those quantities increased, or I might have a small hard drink after the wine. Then, during Lent, I stopped entirely. After Easter, I would drink more for a time, as if I was somehow compensating. And my second blood test was in this post-Lent window. I was drinking more than normal at the time, probably even the evening before the blood test.

In spite of all the facts being before me, I initially failed to make the connection between alcohol and my blood test results. I had not truly accepted alcohol as a carb, which it is, biochemically. It is not glucose, and I was thinking of all carbs as glucose, which activates insulin, and shuts off ketone production. The truth is, I had never looked into the details of how alcohol was metabolized.

Everything came together for me when I delved into the work pediatric endocrinologist Robert Lustig. Every one of his obese patients consumes vast quantities of sugar, and Lustig singles out fructose in particular as the poison responsible for childhood obesity, fatty liver disease, and diabetes. Fructose can only be metabolized by the liver, it readily overloads the liver's mitochondria, and the acetyl-CoA from its metabolism is shuttled directly into fat synthesis, causing high triglycerides, high VLDL, obesity, insulin resistance, and fatty liver disease. Lustig does not distinguish between alcoholic and non-alcoholic fatty liver disease. The symptoms are the same, and the two causes (fructose and alcohol) are metabolized in the same way. I soon found a paper he wrote, where he called fructose, *Alcohol without the buzz*. Some alcohol is metabolized in the brain, which causes intoxication, whereas fructose is not. That is the only metabolic difference of note. Either one will quickly overwhelm the mitochondria, and initiate the same morbid processes. The light finally went on in my head at this point: If, as Lustig said, fructose is as bad as alcohol, then the reverse is also true: Alcohol is as bad as fructose.

Once I saw Lustig's work, my strange results suddenly made perfect sense. I was not eating carbs, but I was drinking alcohol. I lacked glucose, so I was making ketones, but I was also making triglycerides from the excess acetyl-CoA from alcohol metabolism. I now had a clear explanation for my blood profile, but it was not

138

what I wanted to hear: My favorite carb was as bad as fructose, which I considered the worst of the bunch.

Following a festive season, my weight climbs, and my blood glucose tends to also rise. If I bothered with a blood lipid profile, it should only confirm what I already know to be true: I need to correct for the period of excess. And to return to the question I posed earlier: Should I rank the protective properties of elevated HDL above the risk of elevated VLDL? According to the newest version of the lipid hypothesis, elevated HDL should override the risk of elevated triglycerides and VLDL, and there should be no rise in pattern B LDL. But if those lipid factors are only markers of liver stress, then a period of excess alcohol consumption needs to be corrected by a period of abstinence.

How does alcohol fit into our genetic programming, returning to the example of ancient hunger-gatherers? Alcohol was typically only encountered when people ate overripe fruit that had a chance to ferment. This was a sure sign that there was little time left to pile on the pounds, before winter kicked in. And so the body reacts to alcohol exactly as if it was still a signal to pack on those last few pounds. The properties of alcohol are perfectly suited to this purpose. First, it enhances appetite, except in cases of extreme over-indulgence, but such high levels were probably not experienced before our ancestors learned to make their own. Second, alcohol sensitizes the insulin response, thus potentiating all of the anabolic effects of insulin, which means weight gain. And third, alcohol is metabolized by the liver in exactly the same way as fructose. So like fructose, alcohol raises triglyceride levels, leading to elevated VLDL and insulin resistance (the immediate effect of the alcohol is insulin sensitivity, but the longer-term effect of the resulting fat is insulin resistance). If we only consumed alcohol seasonally, there would be no issue. It is the constant availability, and our tendency to over-consume, that poses the biggest risk.

Alcohol is not like glucose, which will put one out of ketosis for several days, because alcohol is not metabolized by any tissue besides liver (and a little in the brain). But it will result in weight gain, and putatively unhealthy blood lipid profiles. The threshold for maxing out the liver's mitochondria, and inducing the toxic properties of alcohol, is thought to be about fifty grams. This may vary between different people, and is also dependent on what else those mitochondria are stuck metabolizing. If the alcohol comes with fructose, for instance, then the effects of the two are additive, and the toxicity threshold drops. So while a shot of vodka, or a glass of dry wine may be okay, a *piña colada* with equal alcohol content is more of a problem. Further, as I learned, a ketogenic dieter who drinks regularly may show an unusual combination of elevated HDL, together with elevated triglycerides and VLDL. This flies in the face of the expectation of an inverse relationship between HDL and triglycerides. The elevated HDL is *probably* the dominant factor in this pairing, but only if the latest iteration of the ever-changing lipid hypothesis is correct. Who wants to be the guinea pig to prove this to be true?

In a previous chapter, I mentioned that Japan and Russia have similar classical risk factors for heart disease, yet Russia has 1,800% more heart disease. I suggested vodka as one big difference, because it stresses the liver, making the liver work overtime to detoxify the alcohol, and turn it into triglycerides. Whether it turns out to be the presence of triglycerides that causes heart disease, or the stress on the liver (I favor that one), it's impossible to ignore excessive alcohol consumption as a risk factor.

I finally decided that regular abstinence is best for me, for several reasons. First, because of the long-term effects on my weight and morning blood glucose. Second, I sleep much better when I'm dry. It may be easier to fall asleep after drinking, but later in the night, the quality of sleep is inferior. If I've drank anything at all, I'll need to go to the bathroom during the night, and often have wakeful spells at 3 am, or so. When dry, it takes a little longer to fall asleep, but I usually sleep all night, and whether I need to go to the bathroom only depends on how much water I drink before bed.

A second distinction should be made between the start of the process of fixing diabetes, versus maintaining it, later. At first, our objective is to break the insulin resistance feedback loop. Second is to reverse the damage done to our livers, and circulatory systems. Most diabetics have accumulated some fat in their livers, so when beginning to put matters straight, it would seem a very good idea to go dry completely. At the minimum, to abstain for one month, after which everyone can judge for themselves whether this all works.

Once a stable weight has been reached, and all symptoms of the transition and hyperglycemia are gone, some amount of occasional alcohol consumption may work, for some people. It depends principally on each individual's ability to restrain himself from over-consumption. My own tendency is that when I am dry, it is easy to stay dry. I sleep better and deeper, and wake feeling far better. Once I open a bottle of wine, I am initially satisfied with a single glass, or maximally two. But after a few days of the same, I start to want more. If a bottle is open, I will want to drain it. That's when I need to break the cycle, and go dry again. What I finally settled on was to open a bottle of wine on Friday and Saturday evenings, and share it. But come the start of the regular week, it is off limits.

Above the toxicity threshold, alcohol is as bad as fructose. I think of them collectively as *fructohol*. Obviously, it is necessary to avoid all sweet drinks, and any all-malt beer, due to its carb content. Various ultra-low carb formulations may possibly be okay within limits, but I dislike them so much, I can't bring myself to look them up ... Okay, okay, I recognize my duty here. I looked them up, and found a few with as little as 2 grams of carb per bottle, which would fit within the same framework as I use for wine. But there's still the matter of the taste. For me, then, beer is strictly off-limits.

It is often said that moderate alcohol consumption is healthy. Those of us who hear that news never forget it, because it legitimizes our enjoyment. But is it true? I have not seen any molecular mechanism by which it could work, nor data to support it. But I also have not researched it exhaustively, so it may be true, we all hope. The best case to be made for moderate social drinking stems from Kendrick's chronic stress model of heart disease development. Moderate drinking, defined as enough to put you in a good mood in the evening, but not enough to spoil your morning mood, can relieve stress. Especially if done socially, with friends or family. It becomes a festive event, and the social element is as significant as the alcohol, or even more so. They key is for it to be occasional, as well as moderate.

I calculated roughly how much one would have to drink to get fifty grams of ethanol, the presumed toxicity threshold. It works out to about three bottles of beer, two thirds of a bottle of wine, or five ounces of spirits. Does this mean it's okay to go that high, but not higher? Not quite. Those are upper limits, but depending on what else the liver is metabolizing, it will usually mean less, and maybe less for women than for men. Will you occasionally exceed this?

Yes, probably. The idea is to let the system recover afterwards, and not do it chronically. Of course, this has nothing to do with legal blood alcohol limits for driving, which are entirely unrelated, and which I do not address.

Summary: Alcohol is metabolized exactly like fructose. Mostly in the liver (and enough in the brain to affect its function, for better and/or worse), and only through the citric acid cycle. Excess amounts go directly into fat synthesis, raising triglycerides and VLDL. Weight gain always follows. I found it useful to go dry initially, to help my liver clear any accumulated fat. Later, I settled on small amounts of wine only on weekends.

Cutting Supplements, Fixing my Vision

I need to stress again that I began this journey with the same preconceived notions most everyone has about insulin resistant diabetes. That the objective is to override insulin resistance, force cells to take up all that glucose, and once accomplished, the problem is solved, or at least stabilized. I never considered that this meant being overweight, hypertensive, and at full diabetic risk of heart disease. I had to learn these things as I went along, and at first, I only wanted to lower my blood glucose, because that is what defines diabetes.

I had already tried metformin briefly, and stopped it when I decided it was making no discernible difference. After a while, I became comfortable with the results I was achieving with the new diet, and medications seemed less and less attractive. I was still experimenting with supplements, but eventually decided many of them were the functional equivalents of drugs, only without patents or a government stamp of approval. I proceeded to cut out any I felt had a pharmacological mode of action, such as corisolic acid, berberine, and cinnamon extract. Cinnamon in the odd food is used sparingly, so it does not cause me any concern. Eventually, I restricted myself to true nutritional supplements and anti-oxidants. And I found no regression in my glucose measurements.

It was in that time frame that I developed the sense that diabetes drugs were shuffling the problem of excess glucose from circulation and into cells. The liver took the brunt. The skit of *Mr. Creosote* from Monty Python's *The Meaning of Life* came to mind at that time. The persistent waiter, forcing the obese man to eat the wafer thin that makes him explode was the equivalent of most diabetes drugs. Even before I reviewed all the mechanisms of insulin resistance, I began to suspect that the latter stages of insulin resistance were a defense mechanism for cells, to protect themselves from the toxicity that was being stuffed into them. It was only as I was finishing this book that I learned that seven multinational, controlled trials of insulin and/or diabetes drugs all failed to reduce the risks of heart disease in diabetics. Some worsened the risks. This appeared to validate my suspicion that liver stress from too much glucose was triggering heart disease.

One of the biggest changes I noticed after reducing my glucose so rapidly was with my vision. Previously excellent, on the order of 20/10, from my mid-40s, I found myself needing reading glasses of increasing strength. It finally reached the point where I began to watch TV with weak reading glasses, of 1.0 diopter. That was a distance of about 12 feet. As my blood glucose fell, and after a short lag time, I suddenly no longer needed glasses for the TV, and reverted to weaker prescriptions for other purposes. Today, I wear 1.0 diopter reading glasses for work on the computer, about 5 feet away. Glucose is an osmotic driver, in that water follows it where it goes. That can swell things, like the lens in the eye, and change its shape.

I do a lot of writing on my computer, and frequently tire my eyes. At one point, I suddenly found a weak double image in my left eye. I tried the various eye tests available online, and it seemed a perfect match for astigmatism, which was something new for me. I could not understand how someone could suddenly develop astigmatism in their fifties. So I got a referral to an ophthalmologist, for a full checkup.

At the ophthalmologist's office, the tests were routine, and he concurred that I had astigmatism, which he said I probably always had, but my eye muscles could compensate when I was younger. He did all the scans of my irises, and the appointment was passing without incident, until I mentioned that I used to be diabetic. He stopped in his tracks, and gave me that now-familiar, quizzical look. *Surely, nobody* used to be *diabetic*. Once you're diabetic, you're always diabetic. He immediately went back, and repeated the same scans on my retinas that he had already done, and initially found no reasons for concern. Now, he pointed to the remnants of some very small hemorrhages, which were probably there on the first scan. "Anything serious?" I asked.

"No, these aren't important" he replied. "But being diabetic, we have to track them more carefully." Lesson one: The medical system will never accept that you're no longer diabetic. It's simply outside the scope of their experience. Lesson two: Given the existing perceptions, they will continue to treat you as a high risk patient.

Measuring Ketones

Nutritional ketosis begins when the levels of beta hydroxybutyrate (BHB) in the blood reach 0.5 mM. Optimal ketosis, from the perspective of weight loss, is a little higher, at 1.5 - 3.0 mM. BHB levels can spike higher than that, to values in the range of 5.0 mM (I've never experienced levels that high), following intensive exercise that mobilizes fat reserves, but then decline within several hours, as trace amounts of insulin signal the liver to stop producing BHB. I rarely find myself exceeding 2.0 mM, and usually measure below 1.5 mM. I have never measured above 3.0 mM, even after exercise.

The easiest way to measure ketones is with the inexpensive urine dipsticks, for as long as they work. Do they turn a robust, purple color? That's ketosis. I expect everyone will start with this assay, due to its low cost and ease of use (you pee on a strip). But it is widely reported that urine ketones tend to disappear after the person becomes fully ketone adapted. In some cases, in only a month or two. And those people often feel discouraged, fearing they've failed to maintain ketosis, when the opposite is often true. For me, it happened between nine and eleven months after I had started. I inferred a loss of ketosis, and at first, attributed it to my dietary and lifestyle slippage, and resolved to improve. Soon, the weight began to come off, but the ketones were gone entirely. What now?

I purchased a breath ketone meter that detected acetone. It is reusable, and requires no expensive consumables, so it was enticing. But I only registered weak ketone numbers, and had a very difficult time trying to estimate my blood BHB from the non-quantitative

144

acetone measurement on the breath meter. I also worried whether breath acetone levels relative to blood BHB levels might change over time, like acetoacetate levels in urine. Clearly, a direct measurement was necessary.

Blood BHB levels are the gold standard of ketosis, and I was already pricking my finger to measure blood glucose, so why not? I have a meter that will measure either glucose or ketones, depending on the strip used. Unlike glucose test strips, which can be had for as little as 13 cents a piece (at publication time), ketone test strips remain expensive. On the order of $1.50 per strip, and that is the lowest price I've managed to find. My first measurement came in at 1.0 mM. I confirmed the absence of ketones in my urine, and found a relatively low measurement with the breath ketone meter. The following day, after my daily walk, I measured 1.9 mM. I was in ketosis after all! Over the following month, I confirmed that there was no good correlation between the blood ketone level and the reading on the breath ketone meter. After establishing this, I decided to keep my testing budget tight, so I only measure my BHB a couple of times a month, depending on when I am curious about the number. The numbers tend to be highest after exercise. A large serving of vegetables is often enough to bring on a reading of less than 0.5 mM, not considered ketosis. I try to strike a balance between eating a rounded diet, and maintaining ketosis. I do not worry that certain meals, if properly nutritious, might lower my ketones for a day or two.

I have not run many consecutive BHB measurements, to establish the accuracy of the strips, but those I have run show a range of about 10%. That's a lot tighter than I expected to see. The strips are designed for those who may worry about ketoacidosis, so they need to discriminate between 1.0 mM and 10.0 mM, not between 1.0 mM and 1.5 mM. The low levels experienced in nutritional ketosis are not considered important. But the way I feel when reading of 1.5 mM is different from a reading of less than 0.5 mM. Ketosis is usually accompanied by a sense of well-being, without feeling in any way impaired. And it tends to agree with what I expect, based on my diet and activity. If I fast, and especially if I fast but for a lunchtime snack of home-made keto friendly chocolate (recipe in Appendix I), my ketones will be substantially higher in the afternoon.

I reiterate that it is not strictly necessary for me to measure my ketones. I am not in any danger of ketoacidosis, and I am going to follow this diet regardless of the reading. But it is validation that I am on the right track. And the confidence that brings can be critical at times, because the medical system will generally not give that kind of affirmation.

Summary: I measure my ketones occasionally, to verify that I'm in ketosis. The easiest way to measure ketones is with urine test strips, but they eventually stop working, as the body adapts. I tried a breath acetone meter, but was not satisfied. In the end, blood ketones are the only good measure.

Exercise and Fasting

Walking is man's best medicine. ~ Hippocrates

As exercise will use up glycogen reserves before switching to fat, one might think that exercise would lower blood glucose levels, right? And it would be true, for people who have not made the adjustment to burning fat. The sluggishness and jitters that afflict many, as their glucose is depleted, is probably also familiar to any diabetic whose glucose drops below recent average levels, even if far above normal. But what happens if the fuel of choice is fat, rather than glucose?

Before I had to confront my diabetes, the duration and difficulty of hikes I could undertake was very limited. My blood glucose would drop, leaving me feeling chronically short of energy. I might even begin to yawn, and feel drowsy. I had to cut those hikes short, because I could not sustain the effort. I could struggle against the headwind, but it would always come much harder for me than it seemed for others.

Then, as I adjusted to burning fat, everything changed. It only took a couple of months for the adjustment to be complete, even if my conditioning continued to improve afterwards. Now, I could walk up a long, steep hill at a steady pace without having to stop, and allow my liver to make more glucose available. I was burning fat, a fuel of which I still had considerable reserves. The rate at which I could exercise was from the outset limited by the fitness of my respiratory system, and the oxygen carrying capacity of my blood. Those continued to improve over time, but the transformation was obvious from the start. Suddenly, hikes of five or more miles, in mountainous terrain, were within my abilities. I'd be sore at the end, but I felt like I could do double the distance, if I had to. My wife had always hiked with me, but as she had not initially adopted my diet, suddenly showed her limitations. She had long had better endurance than me, but now, she was the one who needed a supplementary snack, a source of glucose, to keep her energy up. It did not matter whether I had not eaten anything at all that day. I was nowhere near running out of energy.

So what should I expect of my blood glucose number, after a long hike? In the early days, I would take multiple measurements every day, and reliably found my low for the day to occur late in the afternoon. After the first few months, it would reliably be below 100 mg/dl. So the first time I returned home from a long hike, and found it was time for an afternoon measurement, I was looking forward to seeing a satisfyingly low number. And it came back at 110 mg/dl. *How is that possible?* I wondered. *It was at 98 mg/dl before breakfast, and I haven't eaten a thing since. I've hiked five miles, I'm in ketosis, and yet my glucose is up. Where did it come from?*

Another time, I measured 93 mg/dl on waking. I had a cup of coffee whitened with heavy cream, but no sweeteners. I did not eat anything. I then went for two mile walk, with two significant hills along the way. It's forty minutes of occasionally strenuous walking. I returned, drank a glass of water, and started writing. I measured my glucose again after an hour, and it was 121 mg/dl. Again, I was certain there was no dietary source of glucose. If anything, the fasting compounded the exercise-associated spike in blood glucose.

About a week later, it was early afternoon, and I had not eaten since breakfast. But a shipment of patio furniture arrived, and had to be assembled. The job took me several hours, all of it work with my hands. It was hard work, but not aerobic. I don't believe it raised my breathing rate much, if at all. I thought I even experienced the sensation of low blood glucose, with twitchy eyelids, slight shakiness in the hands, and loss of energy. So after finishing the work, I took a measurement. 120 mg/dl. *What gives?*

Is it stress? Exercise is supposed to reduce stress, right? Well yes, over the long term, or even overnight. But not immediately. Let's be honest, exercise is stressful. If it's good exercise, it's hard work. Your heart and lungs are pushed, and the stress response kicks in. Cortisol is elevated, and blood glucose rises. And for those like me, with apparent defects in the HPA Axis, the stress response is not self-limiting to the same extent as someone without the defect.

If my only objective were lowering my glucose this second, I would sit on the sofa and eat, rather than work myself so hard, or avoid eating, only to find my glucose higher on an empty stomach. But once again, the objective is overall health, and restoration of equilibrium in the long term is more important than a small drop in glucose immediately, if the two are not aligned. And the morning following a long hike, my blood glucose is reliably low. That is the more telling number, and is reflective of the fact that my stress levels have been reduced as a result of the hike, and the rest that followed.

Lastly, my wife's glucose never spikes after exercise, even after adapting to burning fat. She also does not have a morning glucose spike, and those facts together kind of prove she has no defects in her HPA Axis. Fortunately for me, the effect is too small, and brief, to be a serious concern, and does not discourage me from exercise that has long-term benefits.

Summary: Exercise and fasting can raise blood glucose levels in the short term, for someone burning fat. That's not a reason to sit on the couch and eat pretzels and potato chips. The long-term benefits outweigh the short-term costs.

Protein Fasting

One vexing question was whether having been diabetic, I had sustained any permanent damage to my endocrine system. Especially when there were times where my glucose was elevated, I had to wonder whether there was something fundamentally off, that would never recover. To this day, I lack a final answer, but I developed a workable hypothesis. I have sufficient insulin for my needs, and I went from having a gross excess to needing very little. So I don't believe I've had time to damage my beta cells, and that's the principal thing that goes wrong in advanced cases of type II diabetes. What I'm left with is the possibility of epigenetic changes in the regulation of certain genes. The first is glucagon, the hormone that signals the liver to break down glycogen, and once that's gone, to make new glucose from protein. It is made by the alpha cells of the pancreas, which can become insulin resistant. At that point, they produce more glucagon, even in the face of extra insulin. My blood glucose is usually completely normal, so I am probably not chronically over-producing glucagon. But the episodic elevation of my blood glucose suggests something may still be off. It is not from dietary carbohydrates, as I've learned to manage those pretty well. The only remaining possibility is the liver making new glucose, out of protein, in response to cortisol, the stress hormone. And it rises episodically, in response to overall stress.

Can the effects of cortisol be overridden? I'm not talking about stress reduction, exercise, or relaxation. Those can work for a while, but a stress trigger is always right around the corner. What I'm looking for is a trump card, which the stress response cannot overcome.

I believe I found one in the starvation response. I know, I hear you objecting that I've previously said how fasting boosts the stress hormone cortisol, and with it, blood glucose. But the stress response is complicated to the point of strange, in that its long-term effects are often opposite of the short-term. And the principle is simple: Beyond a short fast, the body has to re-order its priorities, in order to survive a possible period of hunger. In the short-term, it boosts glucose by converting protein to glucose. But if it did this indefinitely, it would quicken the depletion of the body's proteins, and hasten death by starvation. Once it realizes protein is in short supply, it has to adapt. And that's what this is: Selective starvation, or the protein fast. Instead of merely eating a high fat, low carb diet with moderate protein intake, one switches to a high fat, low carb, low protein diet. The objective for the duration of the protein fast is to consume less than the body's long-term protein requirement.

The science of fasting is old, and new. It has been around a long time, but enjoys a lot of new interest. Benefits of fasting for extended periods, weeks or even a month, are many. Inflammatory, allergic, other immune dysfunctions, and possibly even cancer, are all greatly improved, or eliminated. In a recent breakthrough, Valter Longo at USC observed that fasted mice treated with lethal doses of a chemotherapeutic agent all survived, while the normally fed controls all died. That observation triggered a flurry of interest, of particular note because people were traditionally told to eat heartily before cycles of chemo. The initial observation seems to be holding up in fasting people, experiencing substantial improvement in both efficacy and toxicity of chemo. Fasting seems to activate a protective response in normal cells, which cancer cells are unable to match.

What I took from these developments is that the body changes its biochemistry when forced to go without food. It decreases gluconeogenesis, and increases fat metabolism for energy. Yes, proteins continue to be broken down to make glucose, but at a reduced rate. And the body also seems to know not to break down all proteins, equally. It seems to pick the old, worn out proteins first. Then, when protein intake is restored, the body restores everything with newly made proteins. It's somewhat rejuvenating.

Once I actually started, I felt some familiar symptoms. On the third day, I felt some nausea, and weakness, which was reminiscent of the adaptation I had to make when cutting out carbs. But it lasted less than a day. I took my regular hour long walk, although it probably took about five minutes longer due to my low energy. By the afternoon, my energy was back.

By the end of the two weeks, my glucose levels were lower, and I have been very resilient in fighting colds since then. It appears to have worked as advertised. I talked my wife into trying it also, and she saw a substantial improvement in allergies that frequently trouble her.

My current plan is to do a twice-annual protein fast of two weeks' duration. For those two weeks, I avoid all meat, and because I do not eat beans or other vegan staples, it is simple to be in a protein deficit. A couple of eggs for breakfast, and some cheese with dinner provide well less than the fifty grams of protein that would be my minimum requirement.

Lastly, protein fasting, by whatever name it is given, is a hot new area of research, so there will be much reported on it in coming years. Stay tuned. I have the feeling we have not heard the last of this topic.

Summary: A useful tool to override the effects of chronic stress is the protein fast. For a limited time, I cut protein intake down as low as reasonably achievable. The body adapts, stops making glucose from protein, and things quickly correct themselves. Then, I restore protein intake to moderate, HFLC levels.

Breaking Ketosis

Occasionally, I've eaten more of something that would have been fine in smaller amounts, and fell out of ketosis. Or unknowingly combined several foods over the course of the day, that in combination, put me out of ketosis. The first thing I always tried to do, once I learned I had lost ketosis, is fast a bit more than normal, and exercise a bit more, to restore ketosis as quickly as I could. If I did things right, I could be back in ketosis in about three days. But remember, if my daily limit is on the order of twenty grams of carb, I might slip and eat thirty grams. Forty at the extreme. But I can be confident I haven't consumed a hundred grams of carbs, let along the three hundred that constitute today's daily recommendations. As a guess, a true carb binge could take a week to work out of the system.

At one point, I stopped to ask whether there may be times when breaking ketosis is a good thing. After everything I've said about insulin, effectively declaring it our biggest health enemy, I am still wedded to the notion that everything physiological exists for a reason. On one hand, insulin resistance is natural. But on the other, it would not be right to never use our insulin response. Put into context, insulin is only our enemy when we over-consume carbs on a chronic basis. But how about episodically? I can think of some exceptions.

The first example is healing. I'm not talking about a simple cut on the skin, but a more serious injury that requires a period of convalescence. Be it surgery, a broken bone, or something equally traumatic. The anabolic properties of insulin are probably not a bad thing at times like that. Muscles and bones heal when stimulated by insulin's close relative, IGF-I (Insulin-like Growth Factor-I), but insulin is also able to stimulate the IGF-I receptor. Parenthetically, growth hormone is secreted in short bursts, stimulates IGF-I production, and then quickly disappears. As an aside, this makes it ideal for athletes who want the benefits of doping, but don't want to get caught. We may look askance at that, and question the damage they are doing to their health. Fair enough, but if the rest of us are doing the same thing all the time with chronically elevated insulin, then let's make it our priority to fix that.

Adolescence is a period of programmed insulin resistance, and also the time when growth hormone does the most work. Most parents know that pre-teens are usually at their chubbiest, but some argue it is important to emerge from adolescence reasonably lean, or lifelong patterns of insulin resistance may become fixed. I don't know if that's true or not, so caution is warranted. I won't let my adolescents binge on too many carbs, simply because it's normal for them to be somewhat insulin resistant at that age.

Another example is sickness. We already discussed how the inflammatory hormones that are the first responders to infection cause elevated glucose levels. They would not do this if the elevated glucose was not useful to the immune system, as it gears up to fight an infection. And at first, when I noticed spikes in my glucose when I was sick, I fought it. I cut back on protein, fasted more, and tried my best to hold my ground. But eventually, I decided to go with the flow. If my body needs the extra glucose to fight a virus, I'll allow if for a day or two. I'll even break ketosis, deliberately.

Does that mean a loaf of bread, a plate of spaghetti, and sugar in the diet? No way. I'm still prone to HPA Axis dysfunction, and the elevated blood glucose and possibly insulin levels that come with it. I have no idea how long it would take for the positive feedback loop to once again spin out of control. I mean something modest. At first, I tried an English muffin with breakfast, and a regular portion of cooked baby carrots with dinner. The English muffin has about 25 grams of net carb, and the serving of baby carrots somewhere around 15 grams. That's enough to put me out of ketosis, but not enough to overwhelm the system. Later, I decided there was something about beans that I occasionally craved. A half cup of those would put me out of ketosis, and satisfy the craving. And not every day, either. I do it as a one-time thing, to give my body the extra glucose it wants, and then revert to carb avoidance. The immune system is fully mobilized within three days, in any case, and I am usually unaware of being sick on day one. So a little extra carb on day two is enough to last until it is fully at work. Once, I had a glucose spike I thought might be the start of a cold, and broke ketosis. But no cold came, so it was probably stress related. Then, something curious happened. I went for my regular 3 mile walk, and about half way through, I suddenly ran out of energy. It was like I hit a wall. This was unexpected, and reminded me of what it was like before I cut carbs. I think my body was burning carbs on that day, and once I ran out, my fat pools were not mobilized quickly enough to make a smooth transition. I dragged myself home, worried what it might be, and rested for another day, back on my low-carb diet. Then I tried it again, and found my energy was back to normal.

How about weight gain? According to the dieting guides, occasionally breaking ketosis, lightly, results in more long-term weight loss than maintaining ketosis, uninterrupted. Clearly, the body needs alternating cycles of building up and breaking down its tissues, to ensure everything is as close to pristine as our age will permit. Lastly, I would never break ketosis with sugar. A little extra glucose may help the immune system fight infection, but fructose only overwhelms the liver's ability to deal with it. It does nothing to boost energy levels, boost the immune system, or provide energy to the muscles.

Summary: If healing from a major injury, or sick, a little glucose may be good. A modest boost is enough to break ketosis. But at all costs, I avoid sugar.

Chapter 8: Tying up Loose Ends

In our society, unless something can be measured then it doesn't exist. This is especially true in the world of medicine. ~ Michael Perkins

Which Is Critical: Eliminating Hyperglycemia, Ketones, or Idling Insulin?

In a hurry to learn the nuances of the ketogenic diet - which has been described in its modern form for some time - I initially took for granted that the presence of the ketone beta hydroxybutyrate (BHB) in the blood was what conferred the benefits attributed to the diet. But in writing this book, I ended up putting a lot more emphasis on breaking the insulin resistance feedback loop. Clearly, reducing the action of insulin to its bare minimum confers many benefits, and eliminating hyperglycemia neutralizes the toxicity of glucose. The presence of blood BHB is an excellent marker of both. They tend to occur together, and ketones will never appear if glucose and insulin are abundant. At this point, it is fair to ask which factors confer which benefit, or whether they are all required. This may seem like an academic exercise, but there is a practical implication. Some people benefit greatly from reducing their carbs, but not to the extent that they produce ketones in their blood. Those people are benefiting from reduced insulin usage, without having blood ketones.

Idling of the insulin response seems to be the principal factor in weight loss, and blood BHB is an indication that fat is being burned, insulin is not in use, and fat cells cannot take up glucose and store fat. The BHB appears to be an associated marker of weight loss, rather than a cause. On the other hand, reports suggest that a diet that boosts ketones is necessary for maximum weight loss. Blogger Jimmy Moore, who lost 180 pounds in a year, subsequently regained over fifty of those pounds, and it took boosting his ketones to again slim down. I believe his body found a way to use its insulin response more efficiently, and defeating it required stronger ketosis. One day, we might learn what effect ten years of ketosis will have on our weight. I'm confident it won't produce ultra-thin people who were previously heavy. But I'm equally confident we will be thinner than before we started.

Improved blood lipid profiles develop when fats are shuttled from fat cells to the liver (HDL), rather than from the liver to fat cells (LDL and VLDL). Likewise, fatty liver disease is eliminated by this reversed flow of lipids. The key is to take the load off the liver, by consuming calories that don't require processing by the liver. In other words, cutting the carbs, and feeding adipocytes directly from the gut. Those adipocytes then send fuel to the liver in HDL particles, which rise to meet demand.

Inflammation is partially responsible for insulin resistance, and so the anti-inflammatory properties of BHB help reverse insulin resistance. Inflammation is also involved in cancer progression, but BHB has additional anti-cancer properties, and research into that topic is currently very active.

How about stress? Stress raises cortisol levels, which primes white blood cells to look for trouble. Another word for that is inflammation. Being in ketosis alone can create a feeling of well-being, but it's not presently clear whether it can prevent stress, or restore HPA Axis function.

Normalization of blood pressure comes from idling the insulin response, as one reverses the chronically elevated insulin levels that caused fluid retention by the kidneys, and overgrowth of vascular smooth muscle. But damage to the microvasculature also has to heal, following the reduction of glucose levels. I know several people who cut their carbs short of producing ketones, but experienced dramatic improvements in blood pressure, and weight loss. They were not diabetic to begin with, but this observation suggests they had chronically elevated insulin, and therefore were somewhat insulin resistant. Their blood lipid profiles also improved dramatically, as the flow of fat reversed.

Summary: Idling the insulin response is the most important thing. Only then can the insulin resistance feedback loop be broken, and blood glucose control can be restored by natural means. The presence of blood ketones is at the least a marker of these things, but also contributes additional benefits on its own.

Trusting How You Feel

The medical system does not trust subjective measures like, "I feel good." I'm sure every good doctor wants his patients to feel good, and the best doctors make a point of getting to know each patient, so they can make an assessment of whether he is *himself*, or somehow off kilter. But most experienced doctors can recall when a patient who always seemed to feel good suddenly keeled over and died. Every patient will eventually die, that's not the issue. It's being surprised by a death that is unsettling to a doctor. So any number that can be plugged into a formula, to spit out a relative risk, gives a doctor some assurance that they've done their job. Even when a low-risk patient dies, if they had a risk score, they can assign any blame to the formula, or attribute it to chance. But to have no parameters representing risk is to feel negligent. *Is there something I could have done?*

To come up with a number representing risk, you need to measure something, and plug that number into a formula. Scientifically trained people are suckers for numbers, and there is no number attached to feeling good, nor any guideline for how good a person is supposed to feel. It's the same as the problem with accepting stress as a cause for disease. Stress has no precise definition, and it would be too much work to develop a numeric one, if it were even possible.

None of this means *we* should underestimate the importance of feeling good, during the course of our every day routine. But we also need to be realistic. I don't expect Monday morning to find you jumping out of bed with a wide smile. But by the time you're at your job and into your routine, it's enough if you don't feel miserable, or excessively tired. If someone walks by and asks a question, can you make it a positive encounter? If you're not feeling good, underneath, it will be hard to offer a smile, and some kind words.

Feeling good means being able to function, in the way you need to, without an underlying health issue getting in the way. It means being able to enjoy leisure activities appropriate for your stage of life and fitness, without being excessively tired. If children or grandchildren need attention at the end of the day, can you give it to them, or are you just too tired?

Insulin resistance gives rise to leptin resistance, which makes you feel lethargic, hungry, and generally *not good*. Reverse leptin resistance, and you end up feeling energetic, and for lack of another

156

word, good. So feeling good is an indication of proper insulin and leptin function. If you feel good, chances are you are not under chronic stress. Your body's functions are in a healthy range, you are not sick, and all those things that can make you feel bad are absent. While feeling good is a worthy goal in itself, its true value is in reassuring you of your overall health. Enter the pharmaceutical mindset: Why not create a drug that makes you feel good? That should make you healthy, right? I'm afraid not. Any drug that could make you feel good by blocking your body's signals to feel bad would only mask what should serve as a warning of an underlying health issue.

With that in mind, a surrogate health marker should not trump how you feel, if there is a conflict between the two. In other words, if you were to feel awful, and fear you might have symptoms of a heart attack or stroke, you don't take comfort in the knowledge that your last A1C measurement was normal, and your cholesterol is low. You get help right away. When my blood glucose was 325 mg/dl, I could not say with any confidence that I felt good. I knew there was something wrong. The glucose reading told me what that thing was, but how I felt should have made me suspect something to begin with. If your blood pressure is truly out of control, you will not feel good. Again, you will know something is wrong. Likewise, if under chronic stress, you feel miserable.

Summary: How you feel matters. Feeling lousy over a long period of time is an indication that something is wrong. Feeling good and energetic is an indication of the opposite.

Frequent Questions

Medical thinking is like a giant ocean liner. Changes in direction happen slowly, and face much resistance. When everything is going well, that is understandable. You don't want to veer off in all different directions, if you're heading the right way. But what about when there's a shoal ahead? Or if we want to scale the problem to be proportional to the size of the diabetes epidemic, we would have to make that shoal the size of a continent. Life expectancy in the West is now dropping, and most of it is due to the complications of diabetes. Clearly, there are times when the ocean liner has to execute extreme maneuvers, or face disaster.

The metaphor of the ocean liner represents medical thinking on the question of how extreme a dietary change is needed to break the feedback loop of insulin resistance. On one hand you have my experience, which was that of success with an extreme change. I represent only one data point, but it's an important data point. It was a success, which proves it possible to beat diabetes with a dietary change, and without drugs. Yet medical thinking is not comfortable with drastic change, so it will reflexively argue for a more modest change. This may create some conflict between doctor and patient, and test the patience of both. My only advice is to hold all advice accountable. Results are what matter, and if doctor-mandated modest change does not achieve them, then it's not enough. Until the majority of doctors see their diabetic patients cure themselves, they will be skeptical it can even work. Makers of diabetes drugs will not send their sales reps with cartoon brochures touting the HFLC diet. If anything, they will sneer at it, because of the threat it poses to drug sales. So it's up to us diabetics, to turn the ocean liner with the power of our results.

One question I get quite often is some version of, "What does this diet mean, in practice? Do I have to give up ... ?" What follows is a list of that person's favorite foods, or beverages. "Could I refrain at intervals, and indulge less regularly?" Sweet desserts come up a fair bit. Beer is up there, also. My answer is generally that while a young, healthy person will benefit from even modest reductions in carb consumption, once diabetes has set in, a mere reduction will probably not break the positive feedback loop of increasing insulin resistance. At most, it will slow its progression. But I qualify this opinion by noting it *is* an opinion, and not an empirically established fact. For any given person, it's their glucose meter that will provide the definitive answer.

Next question: *After I break that feedback loop, can I return to the way I used to eat?* For me, the way I used to eat made me diabetic. Under no circumstances will I risk it again, and I can't in good conscience tell anyone else to revert, either. Diabetes may not return immediately, but that person is already known to be susceptible.

Okay, let's back up a step. Let's say I had clued in when I noticed sugar-coma in my late twenties, and incorporated episodes of low-carb eating. I could have gone a few months without carbs, and reset the system to factory specifications. Could I then eat carbs like before? The answer is *probably yes*, for some period of time. How long a time, I can't answer. Blood insulin levels are not routinely measured, but that measurement would be very useful to young people. High insulin levels are a hallmark of the developing feedback loop, and breaking it early and regularly should make for huge health gains later in life. This one measurement at a young age, and a corrective diet to fix elevated insulin, could save the medical system unimaginable amounts of money, and the patients, needless morbidities. I call on all medical professionals to take note.

Does everyone have to ditch the carbs? For once, I am able to say no. First of all, everyone is free to do what they want, and nobody has to copy what I did. Athletes who routinely deplete their glycogen reserves can eat carbs with little harm. The traditional Japanese rice farmer or fisherman, whose physical activity was enough to keep the system in balance, and lived longer than us in the West, obviously did not need my advice. But while he ate rice, he did not consume refined sugar, and I think that's significant. Next are people who for cultural or religious reasons fast regularly. They are going to have a degree of resistance to diabetes. A once-a-week fast will deplete glycogen reserves, and may prevent the feedback loop from ever setting in. This tactic may be an excellent approach for young people who do not want to cut out carbs altogether. And there may be others who for genetic reasons are better able to cope with carbs. For many, episodic carb avoidance will be enough. But for diabetics, there is no other viable solution. Pumping the glucose into cells does not solve the problem.

It is emotionally difficult for me to speak to a diabetic who refuses to change his or her diet. "I can't give that up," is something I often hear. The temptation for a doctor in that situation is obviously to write a prescription and be done with it, but it should be with the knowledge that heart disease risk will not decline, and may even increase. And while the conversation may be difficult, the logic is not. If the patient wants to fix the downward health trend, a radical dietary change is essential.

I once had a question about a third person with advanced diabetes. He was interested in my diet, and assumed there was some secret gimmick behind it. He loves cakes, desserts, and other forbidden foods. Could he continue with these, yet conform to the diet? My reply was that if he was not willing to let those go, without exception, there was no point discussing it any further. If it seems like I was being harsh, it is because I know HFLC works, while gimmicks are not known to work. Until another regimen is shown to work, I will not endorse it on the hope that it *might* work.

The model I proposed, of a natural positive feedback loop spinning out of control, explains why diabetes is so common in our carb-rich environment, and why I was able to reverse it so quickly. Once the hurricane of diabetes runs ashore, it is deprived of further fuel (carbs), and quickly dissipates. I predict it necessary to starve the insulin response, in order for insulin levels to fall, and for insulin resistance to disappear. This is accompanied by weight loss, reduced blood pressure and reduced inflammation. But it can't begin until all glucose and glycogen reserves are used up. If I were to guess, I'd say something like 90% of the benefit comes from the last 10% of effort, and I have difficulty imagining a moderate carb reduction achieving that final 10%. My hypothesis argues that diabetics need the full effort, to break the vicious feedback loop of insulin resistance.

In summary, I believe that diabetics must be strict about avoiding carbs, to the point that they produce ketones. Some may suggest otherwise. So is this one of those myriad medical questions, where you consult ten doctors and get eleven opinions, leaving you more confused than ever? It need not be so, and nobody needs to trust my opinion. All I suggest is you conduct your own trial, of n=1. The result of that trial is far more important to you, than to anyone else. It is about your health, and is not simply another data point. In one month, it should be obvious whether it has worked, and I'm highly certain it will work, if you eliminate carbs entirely. I don't know what will happen if done in moderation.

Summary: To properly starve the insulin response, it's probable that carb consumption must be eliminated, at least for a time. 90% of the benefit comes from the last 10% of effort. After that, I can't say whether some amount of regular carb consumption will be okay. I occasionally break ketosis, but barely and rarely. I won't risk going back to the way I was.

How Hard is the Change?

The simple answer is, it's simple. You just stop eating all carbs, and substitute fatty alternatives. That's not the hard part. It's a little harder to deal with some of the carb cravings at first, but those go away, with time. The most important thing is to learn to eat satisfying foods, so you never have to leave the table hungry.

The challenge is to maintain it over time. Social situations are always problematic. I suddenly noticed that any company picnic, church social, or informal get-together was literally a carb-feast. I have yet to see a single invitation to a high fat low carb fundraising event. It is always spaghetti or donuts. More often than not, I make a donation, but skip the event. And this can make you feel isolated, or that the sponsors of those events are insensitive to your needs. You end up cooking at home an awful lot. You will pore over restaurant menus with carb-o-phobia. You'll pick the fattiest cut of meat, and even then, limit yourself to between three and four ounces.

That aside, once you settle into your new routine, it's not bad at all. You'll douse meat in a buttery or creamy sauce, and always leave the table satisfied, yet never bloated. You won't need a nap after eating, and will be able to complete a strenuous workout a half hour after dinner. You will experience *zero* spike in blood glucose after a meal, and you'll feel very satisfied about what you've accomplished. But there will be sacrifices, and you will miss some of your old favorites. For the first year or so, I literally dreamed of a good rye bread. I now have a good bread recipe, and many other low-carb alternatives (Appendix I).

Now, it is time for some specifics. For starters, how to eliminate carbohydrates, which are hiding under every rock.

Avoid:

- Sugar of any type (yes, even if it's *organic*, and even honey, and agave) in coffee, tea, or any beverage. Careful, there are at least 56 different names that mean *sugar*. Look at the nutrition label, not the ingredients list

- Any standard dessert. You'll have to make alternative ones yourself

- All fruit juices (even if they say *no sugar added*. There's plenty that comes from the fruit)

- *Naturally sweet* things, including many fruits. I reiterate, it does not matter where the sugar comes from. Grapes are probably the worst, while wild berries are the safest fruit. But even there, use moderation

- Ketchup, Barbecue Sauce, any other sweetened marinade or condiment

- All *Americanized* Chinese food. Certainly every Chinese buffet I've ever visited in the US or Canada. Everything has a sweet glaze, or sauce. I'm not familiar with authentic Chinese food, so my only comment is that rice is out

- Energy bars, fiber bars, nearly every other snack bar. Even the so-called *Cave Man Bars* are sweetened with sugar. They simply call it something else

- Granola, all cereals, oatmeal, and grains

- Potatoes, Rice, Bread. Any other starchy side to a meal

- Pasta of any type

- Anything made of flour, or with flour

- Battered or breaded foods (after much experimentation, my wife and I found an excellent alternative, see Appendix I)

- Conventional Pizza. Alternative crusts are possible.

- Beer. For those whose tastes accommodate the various ultra-light formulations, there may be a little wiggle room. For me, there is none

- Any sweetened liquor or liqueur. Any sweet wine.

The list is probably not even inclusive. It is probably essential to avoid any kind of boxed food, because everything is formulated with carbs and/or sugars. One has to learn to read nutrition labels, and ignore ingredient lists, because they often confuse the issue with misleading names. It even strikes me as deliberate. Who calls sugar, *organic dehydrated cane juice concentrate*? That's like calling water, *oxide of two single-proton atoms*. What's the point, except to deceive? So go straight to the nutrition label, and look for the net carbs. Fiber is technically a carb, so subtract that from total carbohydrates for net carb content. And sugars are listed separately, a useful thing.

Supplement Facts

Serving Size: 1 Bar (45 g)

Servings Per Container: 1

	Amount Per Serving	%DV
Calories	140	
Calories from Fat	35	
Total Fat	4 g	6%
Saturated Fat	1.5 g	7%
Trans Fat	0 g	
Cholesterol	0 mg	0%
Sodium	80 mg	3%
Total Carbohydrate	32 g	11%
Dietary Fiber	12 g	48%
Soluble Fiber	8 g	
Insoluable Fiber	4 g	
Sugars	11g	
Other Carbohydrate	9 g	
Protein	3 g	
Vitamin A 0%		Vitamin C 0%
Calcium 6%		Iron 8%

*Percent Daily Values (DV) are based on a 2,000 calorie diet.

Here's an example of a nutrition label I took from a box of snack bars. Each bar has 32g of total carbohydrate, but 12g of fiber, for net carbs of 20g. Off limits for me. Of the 20g of net carbs, 11g are sugars, probably split between glucose and fructose, leaving 9g as starches. Needless to say, I no longer buy these bars.

That aside, the news is mostly good. You won't be eating tofu and kale, with an occasional splurge of olive oil drizzled on the top (unless of course you want to. In that case, use a lot of fatty dressing). There are many, highly satisfying ways to eliminate carbs. It only takes a bit of adjustment. By substituting vegetables for starchy sides, you might even end up eating more varieties of vegetable. The number of available low-carb alternative foods is quite extensive, and many low-carb recipe books are available. My approach was to find a way to substitute the carb heavy ingredients in my favorite meals, to adapt them to my needs. In most cases, what emerged was a superior tasting, and satisfying product. I'm still learning of new ones, but those I have at press time are presented in Appendix I.

There is plenty of science that supports this approach, even if going against everything we've been led to believe for those decades can at first be frightening. Even the ketogenic diet books were not enough to prepare me for what I, as a diabetic, would face. But it was definitely worth it. If I was tested for the first time today, the doctor would not know I was ever diabetic. And that makes everything worthwhile.

Summary: There are forbidden foods, and restaurants are a hassle. But I found the low carb alternatives satisfying, and more nutritious than starchy sides.

Three Years Out

Depending on my stress levels, my glucose is sometimes absolutely normal, and sometimes a little elevated. If it's an extended stressful period, my weight will even climb a bit. A protein fast will fix it quickly enough. I don't know if my HPA Axis will ever recover, or if I'll be stress prone for the rest of my life. I'm prepared to accept the latter, even if I hope for the former. At least when I measure my morning glucose, I have a formal reminder that I need to reduce my stress, if the number comes back a little elevated, and I'm not coming down with a cold. Likewise after a festive season. A little more drinking and feasting, and the glucose number will remind me to make a correction.

I continue to measure my glucose every morning, but so long as I stay with the low-carb diet, I do not consider it essential. When I travel, I don't normally bring a glucose meter, since I have limited control over my diet. It's far more important to avoid carbs and sugars as much as possible, limit alcohol consumption, and keep my weight under control. I exercise regularly, usually every day, but I no longer stress over it if I have to miss a day or two.

Low carb life (Jimmy Moore calls it *livin' la vida low-carb*) still poses some challenges. Restaurants are always tense places for me, for instance. One day, my wife wanted to take the kids to the Broken Yolk, a chain that specializes in egg based dishes, assuming I should be able to find something acceptable. Well, it still required a special order to ensure that sides loaded with starch or sugar were kept off my plate. Then, when my omelet arrived, it was missing all the fat that I make sure to drip on to the plate, be it butter or bacon fat, when I cook at home. They probably drained it all away, thinking they were doing their customers a service. But without the fat, I was still hungry after eating. Jimmy Moore writes that he always asks for a large plate of real butter at a restaurant, and I think that's a good idea. But be careful. Butter is more expensive than trans-fat based margarine, and restaurants are always looking to save money.

My father, who was initially skeptical of any dietary solution to diabetes, is now a convert, and has discovered he does not need nearly as much insulin when he reduces his carb load. His liver is probably healthier, also.

In terms of my other symptoms, my blood pressure is under control, usually below 130/80. But this can change very quickly. For instance if I were to take a phenylephrine decongestant, it would spike above 160 for several days. Or if I drink too much, over the course of several days, it will rise more gradually. But in both cases, removal of the offending cause will normalize it quickly enough. I have not taken blood pressure medication for some time. The tingling in my toes has subsided, and is only rarely noticeable today. Blisters or scrapes on my feet now heal normally. I feel like I am in better health than I have been in my adult life. And I was largely ignorant of the question in childhood, so it is safe to say I have never felt better, had better endurance when exercising, or more energy for everyday tasks. I had my heart checked twice over the course of my recovery, and both times it came back perfectly healthy. Given how fearful I was three years ago, I'll take that, gratefully.

Cost of Healthcare

The public blabbers about preventive medicine, but will neither appreciate nor pay for it. You get paid for what you cure. ~ Martin H. Fischer

If doctors conducted research, attended seminars, wrote papers, and other activities in addition to seeing patients, they could devote more time to independent thought and inquiry. They would not depend exclusively on the drug reps for their continuing education, and would know the flaws in the cholesterol hypothesis. That would free them to recommend the HFLC diet as the obvious cure for diabetes. But it's a given they could not see as many patients. With the current configuration of the health care system, that would not work. But is that because of the doctors themselves, or the way health care is administered? After all, interventions are the real cost drivers.

When medicine intervenes, and saves the life of a young or middle-aged person, who then enjoys a normal life expectancy, we all applaud. That's what we want from our medical system. Those types of maladies are typically acute. In other words, you notice something is wrong, you see the doctor, and he fixes it. Next we have the gray area of preventive screening. Some forms of screening may be worthwhile, but too often, screening guidelines are driven by the supply of interventions and screening techniques, rather than the demand of a disease. Lastly, there's the biggest cost driver: The constant monitoring of every fart from a diabetic, and treatment of all the complications of diabetes.

This brings us to costs, which we all pay in some form or other. In the United States, health insurance is paid jointly by employers and employees. The costs are felt directly, leading many to prefer universal health insurance through the government, which is not free, either. The money spent on healthcare is not available for other things, from salary, if an employer is paying the bill, to additional benefits/lower taxes, if paid by government. The costs have escalated so far that everything else is squeezed by the cost of health care. But debating the best way to fund the current healthcare system would divert attention from the salient point: Any way a society chooses to pay for health care as it exists today, the system costs too much. And diabetes is the single biggest driver of those costs.

166

It is useful to imagine what alternative scenarios could play out when someone like me comes into the doctor's office for the first time, with a diagnosis of diabetes. In the established version of how it works, I would be given drugs for blood glucose, hypertension and cholesterol, and sent to specialists to monitor my heart, feet, kidneys, retinas, and whatever else is considered a possible risk. Continuing on this path for many years, the complications from diabetes will worsen, and I may undergo major hospitalizations for any of: Heart attack, stroke, kidney disease, limb gangrene, or cancer. Until my death, every step along that path racks up huge bills for me and the health care system. It no exaggeration to imagine it costing in excess of a million dollars per diabetic. With a third of all Americans now diabetic or pre-diabetic, that represents 100 million people, each costing one million dollars. It's easy to miss how many zeros are actually in the final number. The total bill is *one hundred trillion dollars*! I hope it's obvious to everyone that this is not sustainable.

The alternative possibility, when I present myself at the doctor's office, is that I'm told to cut out carbs, and exercise. To break the insulin resistance feedback loop. The symptoms of diabetes fade, my health improves, and tests are not done if they will not change the way I manage my health. I hope to live longer, in better health, and yet cost the system very little. Ideally, my children will eat differently, and never become diabetic. Doctors can see more different patients, because they will have fewer visits with me. They might even have time for independent inquiry, and if the cost per visit rises, it would still be spread over more people, so every person's total bill would be lightened, and some of the money saved could help those remaining people with chronic health issues. Prescription drug spending would plummet, and most of the current health care cost crisis would disappear, even while life expectancy recovers its recent losses. The burden on the system would be so much lighter that the question of how the bills are paid would be less important. That is what I'd like to see happen, and what I am trying to do with my own life.

Chapter 9: The Revolution

The patient has the right to accept your advice or to ignore it. ~ Martin H. Fischer.

Here is the introductory sentence from a paper with 27 authors, all of whom are credentialed scientists, medical practitioners, or both (Feinman et al., Nutrition 31:1-13, 2015).

> *The inability of current recommendations to control the epidemic of diabetes, the specific failure of the prevailing low-fat diets to improve obesity, cardiovascular risk, or general health and the persistent reports of some serious side effects of commonly prescribed diabetic medications, in combination with the continued success of low-carbohydrate diets in the treatment of diabetes and metabolic syndrome without significant side effects, point to the need for a reappraisal of dietary guidelines.*

This begs the question: If the guidelines were indeed reappraised, would the new guidelines be any better? Most of the information we have today was available in the 1970s, but was ignored. How do we know it would not be ignored again, today? The other factor is time. The diabetes epidemic is out of control, and if we wait another five years for new guidelines to emerge, the costs might be too high to bear. For any given diabetic, those costs are personal.

In the 1970s, we were asked to cut dietary fat from 40% to 30% of total calories. As a people, we complied. The results? The recent *US Centers for Disease Control and Prevention's National Diabetes Statistics Report* states that 30 million Americans have full blown diabetes, while 80 million have pre-diabetes, which typically turns to full blown diabetes within five years. Put another way, a third of all Americans are either diabetic or pre-diabetic. A full 25% of those over the age of 65 have full blown diabetes, and the incidence of diabetes has tripled since 1980. And these numbers will quickly become obsolete, as the picture is looking worse all the time. Obesity and heart disease rates have likewise skyrocketed. Stress plays a role, and always did, but I don't believe a new stress epidemic exploded in 1980.

Back to the guidelines. We, the people, did our part. Did we get what we were promised? By now, the answer should be clear. The guidelines stand at odds with the Hippocratic principle to do no harm, and now it's time to hold those guidelines accountable.

Accountability

When we give government the power to make medical decisions for us, we in essence accept that the state owns our bodies. ~ Ron Paul

This discussion began with the unique circumstances under which our ancestors encountered rich sources of carbohydrate. They always came immediately before a season of hunger, and insulin resistance in muscles was a handy way to divert glucose from muscles to the liver, for fat production. Of course, today's situation is vastly different. Carbohydrates are plentiful at all times. And yet the program hard-wired in our genes has not changed. Without the abrupt, annual disappearance of carbohydrate, the positive feedback loops spins out of control. Obesity and/or diabetes result. And the medical system's answer?

To the obese: "Don't eat so much. Eat whole grains." Have you ever tried to find true whole-grain products that are not fortified with sugar, molasses, or HFCS? I'm not convinced they even exist, although I no longer look for any grain products. And to diabetics: "Take our expensive drugs, and force-feed ever more glucose to your cells." But cells can't handle a chronic excess of glucose any better than the blood can. So forcing ever more glucose into those cells is a recipe for increased insulin resistance and heart disease.

Diabetes is very different from something like an acute heart attack, which is a low-frequency, high-consequence event. What makes diabetes unique is the ease with which one can track progress from day to day, and month to month. Because of the ease with which blood glucose can be monitored, it is also possible to judge, in a short period of time, whether any given treatment is working. Armed with this information, we diabetics can ignore all the so-called *expert* advice, which brought us to the present diabetes epidemic. And just as the patient is entitled to pass judgment on bad advice, the medical professional should also respect results, rather than guidelines. Thirty days is enough time to know if something is working, including a HFLC diet. If it fails, please reject it, and condemn this book. But on the other hand, give logic a chance. The sanctioned advice has produced the opposite of what we wanted, so try the opposite of the advice. Cut out all carbs, and satisfy your hunger with fat. Learn for yourself if poisoning by excess carbohydrate can't be solved by cutting out dietary carbohydrates. A complete cure may take up to ninety days, but thirty days is long enough to get a good idea if it is working. What do you have to lose by trying it for a month, and then passing judgment?

Embracing Dissent

Before a widespread error can be corrected, it must be permissible to question it. Obvious as that sounds, those in positions of influence do not take kindly to being questioned, contradicted, or worse. This is to be expected, and the people should understand that establishing the truth will always be a battle. What I did not expect, and yet found common, is the extent to which those who dissent from orthodoxy are shunned by all the traditional gatekeepers of the scientific establishment. Publishers, journalists, pundits and politicians instinctively adhere to what is perceived as correct, and ignore or attack those who challenge it.

William Banting was widely attacked for spreading news of his personal success losing weight. Robert Atkins was despised by the medical establishment. News coverage of his diet was never objective, and his own publishers are said to have made him de-emphasize the importance of fat in the diet. Clearly, it was not permissible to question the reigning recommendations to reduce fat intake. And yet, it is the ability to think critically, unclouded by self-interest and especially self-justification, that defines an independent thinker. It requires the embrace of dissent and disagreement, especially where a pet theory is concerned. When people are condemned for questioning orthodoxy, the collective wisdom of the society suffers. We all get self-righteous when reminded of how Galileo was treated, yet we're quick to join the modern inquisitors who shout down dissenters from today's orthodoxies. "But I only shout it down when it's wrong," is the inquisitor's reply. Of course, that inquisitor starts by deciding what is right or wrong, and that decision informs what ideas, data, and even people, are acceptable. It is exactly backwards to how science is said to work, and it's a perfect description of how the establishment treats any dissident who cannot be ignored.

170

Admittedly, dissidents have a way of getting under people's skin. Unless they're confrontational, it's too easy to ignore them, so they ramp it up to where they get noticed. Galileo and Copernicus pursued the same idea, but Copernicus was tolerated, while Galileo was censured. The difference? Copernicus was polite, and only put forth an idea that could be ignored. Galileo proved it, and shouted it out for all to hear. Looking back, it's easy to see how it doesn't do science or society any good to judge people and ideas this way. Wrong ideas should be proven wrong, rather than shouted down, with a refusal to even consider them. Otherwise, we build new errors on top of old ones, with ever worse consequences.

Of course, medicine reflects and contains of all of the above dysfunction, with the added layer of lots of money at stake. In medical schools, every professor teaches the cautionary example of Ignaz Semmelweis, who proved that if doctors disinfected their hands before giving obstetric exams to new mothers, they could drastically reduce deaths by septicemia. His proofs were rejected by the medical establishment, and he was committed to an insane asylum, where he soon died. But those same professors then turn around and obstinately defend today's medical errors, especially if their own practice can be called into question. Medical residencies, the equivalent of apprenticeships, are where such conformity is institutionalized. The stories from junior residents who carelessly suggest the senior professor is wrong, and barely make it out alive, are legion.

Today's errors are more numerous than ever, simply because everything has become so standardized, with guidelines covering everything. In a dispute, a doctor knows he will be judged by his adherence to those guidelines. Individual doctors have far less discretion to think for themselves, and in any case, little time to do so. All medical decision making power thus is being centralized in the committees that formulate guidelines. Those on such committees typically have no skin in the game, yet they hold outsized power over the public health, for good or ill. For me and so many others, it was for ill.

Conspiracy Time

We'll know our disinformation program is complete when everything the American public believes is false. ~ William Casey, former CIA Director

Casey probably made that statement in the context of a Cold-War strategy to mislead the Soviet Union, so it's best not to take it as a smoking gun, proving malice in office. But spend ten minutes on the internet, and you'll find dozens like it. And the sentiment they express makes for a useful opening to this section, where we ask how it's even possible to be so wrong, for so long, without actively wanting to be.

Was it an honest mistake, that the official dietary advice was the exact opposite of what is healthy? That it persisted for so long, in the face of logic and evidence as skewed as it is, makes people eventually shrug, and wonder what really goes on behind closed doors. I was long reticent to speculate on the matter. I would prefer the question be directed to those who made the recommendations. I am only one of a hundred million or so in America who suffered the effects of the advice. But few of those originally involved in creating the recommendations are still alive. While he was alive, Ancel Keys could have shed light on his motives, but he never did.

Keys quickly won the backing of the establishment. Why was this, when no solid scientific case was ever made? Was it because the advice that came from it, to avoid meat and eat grains, was in line with environmental and/or animal rights concerns? Those are probably factors today, but the medical bias against animal fats has existed since William Banting's day, before modern sensibilities took shape. But it is undeniable that Keys was the first to propose a narrative that claimed to explain heart disease. Having that narrative, scientists could judge the validity of data, based on whether they were in agreement with Keys' model. Those who disagreed were wrong, and could be ignored. Those who disagreed too loudly were obviously corrupt, and needed to be silenced. Gary Taubes' chronicle of the development and compounding of so many errors (*Good Calories, Bad Calories*) does an excellent job of showing how the lethal combination of science, the political process, a lot of arrogance from both, and herd-following by everyone else, led us into the present mess.

Science is always short of quality data, and overwhelmed with questionable data. That is especially true of the epidemiology of a chronic disease. To treat all data equally, when there is no obvious pattern in sight, would tie your brain into knots. It is therefore overwhelmingly tempting to latch on to a narrative, to use as a filter. It is what Sherlock Holmes warned about, and it's the principal source of error in science. When the issue at hand affects public health, the problem is amplified by the people's hunger for an answer they can embrace.

Once a narrative was in place, it was too late for actual data to make a difference. Keys' appearance on the cover of *Time*, together with the proclamation of his saturated fat hypothesis as the victor, made him a legend in his field. Open disagreement with his ideas became untenable. It takes someone of extraordinary stature to challenge a powerful orthodoxy. Everyone else is cowed into silence, or shouted down as dangerous, if they ramp up the intensity of their dissent.

Then, public policy becomes involved. A public platform is put forth with great fanfare, supported by an emergent consensus among hand-picked scientists. Dissenters are ignored and vilified, because entertaining dissent would only undermine the message, and undercut the case for immediate action. Public policy picks winners, and money follows. Those industries that emerge as winners formally embrace the process, to ensure their advantages are institutionalized. Foods declared to be healthy make it into school and poverty programs, and receive subsidies. The food industry quickly adapts, and advertises their compliance with guidelines as a selling point. "Low-fat" is on the front of the box, in big letters. "High carb" has to be inferred from the small print, on the nutrition label. Any uncertainty that prevailed in the early days is eventually forgotten, as few holdouts remain who were not educated in the prevailing paradigm.

The politicization of science eventually distorts the science so completely that the original error is enforced as dogma even over other fields, who are pressured to base every piece of their own advice on the original error. The American Diabetes Association continues its slavish adherence to the saturated fat-heart disease link, so much so that it recommends a low-fat, high-carb diet for diabetics. They cite no evidence to support any benefits, or even attempt to explain why throwing gasoline on the fire is supposed to lessen the severity of the flames. Conformity to the message is valued above the truth, as those now in positions of authority have no interest in questioning orthodoxy. To do so would jeopardize their positions.

Today, the cracks in the dam are visible, and growing. The errors of the current paradigm have grown too massive to ignore. But what solution is offered up, to fix the problem created by the combination of complex epidemiological science and politics? More combinations of science and politics, only this time with smarter and/or more honest people steering the process (which translates as those currently in leading positions, rather than those who held those positions at a previous time). Do I have a better idea? It would be arrogant of me to assert anything like that. I will settle for taking back the trust we have given to a system that does not merit that trust. To judge for ourselves what works.

What is To Be Done

The first duty of the physician is to educate the masses not to take medicine. ~ William Osler

This is where you often see the author's ideas about changing the scientific and political processes, with the promise of a better outcome. That's not in my nature. Any process that would be tasked with altering the dietary recommendations is a successor of the same process that developed them, and would be prone to the same basic dysfunction. In a pluralistic society, every interested party gets to have their say. And the outcome is an attempt to appease the largest numbers, often skewed to the most influential. If a new process were convened, chances are new errors would be enshrined, and the new recommendations would be no more trustworthy than those of today. I would rather there be no formal recommendations at all, if only to satisfy Hippocrates' admonition to *first, do no harm.* Put another way, *no advice* is always better than *bad advice.* And our diets were far healthier before we were advised how to eat.

Any meaningful change has to come from the grass roots. People who take ownership of their own health, working with their doctors, and judging what actually works. People who measure their glucose, and judge recommendations based on their results. Can you eliminate diabetes drugs with the latest advice? If not, the advice is wrong. Time to move on to something else. The measuring stick for good advice is whether a message is accepted, and spreads. In a three years, I have seen a substantial acceleration in the acceptance of the low-carb message. Low-carb diets are an obvious thing for diabetics to try, and many already have. I have converted, directly or as converts of converts, dozens of people to low-carb eating (counting only those I know about). Some of them were not diabetic, but suffered other effects of Carb Disease, aka Metabolic Syndrome.

Society will change once enough of us demand that it changes. Less with our voices than with our dollars. Every HFLC convert now shops differently. They no longer buy the food products that harm them. They too bypass the processed food aisles in grocery stores. They withhold their dollars from makers of the offending items. And I am certain this will be noticed, if it has not already been noticed. Nothing drives change in corporate attitudes faster than a falloff in sales. But it goes beyond the grocery store. If I find a restaurant with a HFLC-friendly menu (less rare all the time), I compliment them on it. If they do not, I sometimes try to let them know they should serve this growing segment. Good restaurants, and even good fast food chains, listen to customer feedback, knowing that one person saying something equals one hundred thinking it. But my biggest source of encouragement is knowing the truth, when validated by personal experience, rather than being proclaimed by a technocrat, is inherently viral. It spreads without coercion, taxes, or regulations. The critical element is seeing a personal benefit. If a message is preachy, or if it doesn't respect the intelligence of the people, it is rejected. But if done in a helpful way, friend to friend, advice is accepted, especially when it leaves a trail of success in its wake. The person adopting it sees a benefit in short order, and then becomes an advocate to others, ensuring the continued spread of the truth.

For some time, I wrestled with the question of how I can guarantee I'm right, and others are wrong. You will undoubtedly come across conflicting advice, so how are you supposed to know who, and what, to believe? What finally settled the issue for me was recalling that in spite of starting out ignorant of many important facts, I had reduced my own blood glucose from 325 mg/dl to under 150 mg/dl in my first three weeks of trying. And within three months, I had definitively broken the insulin resistance feedback loop, and left diabetes behind. It's results that matter, not credentials or finely stated arguments. Who are you going to believe, the face on TV with the bow tie and rumpled tweed jacket with patches on the elbows, telling you how to eat, or your glucose meter?

If I'm lucky and am not simply ignored, my experience will be panned as only *anecdotal* evidence. They'll say what really matters are large, randomized trials, conducted and analyzed by experts, with a final set of recommendations endorsed by a blue ribbon panel. To which I say that if they had run proper trials before formulating the present guidelines, this discussion would not have been necessary. And I hold a trump card: My one data point is the one that matters to me. I know what I've lived through, and no blue ribbon panel can take that away from me. And the same applies to every diabetic. Nobody else cares for your health as much as you do. Take ownership, and ask yourself whether the guidelines are working. Have they produced weight loss, reduced blood pressure, and controlled blood glucose, without drugs? Have they made you healthy, able to exercise intensely, and feel good overall? Do you expect it to reduce your risk of heart disease, in the face of seven large trials that have failed to do that? Or do they point the finger back at you, for a lack of compliance with their unrealistic guidelines?

When held to account, the HFLC diet came out a resounding success, for me, and for many others. So run your own, short trial: Thirty days on a strict low carb, moderate protein diet, using extra fat (butter, sour cream, cheese, or a fatty sauce of your creation) to satisfy your hunger. After that, you will be able to pass judgment on the results of this advice, versus the track record of the current guidelines. Has your glucose dropped significantly? I'd be shocked if it did not. You're not adding any through your diet. Have you lost weight? Of course you have. You've shut off the insulin signal that's been driving you to put on weight. Those who are not diabetic will see an immediate improvement in their blood pressure. Diabetics will have to be more patient, as the dual effects of smooth muscle cell hypertrophy, and deterioration of the microvasculature

176

correct themselves. But that too will come, with time.

So cut out the carbs, and keep track of your glucose numbers. If you have more questions, browse the books and videos I mentioned throughout, so you hear the full story about fat, cholesterol, and ketones. It is important to develop personal confidence in your new lifestyle, because the medical system will not be supportive. Then, after a month, compare the results, before and after. Did you see the same dramatic improvements I did? Consider making the change permanent. Why would you want to go back to the way it used to be?

If you feel moved to share your results, please do so on the Amazon review page. Let others see whether this advice is worthwhile, or not. The only value of advice is in what it can do for you. If it passes that test, then we need not concern ourselves with the guidelines. The truth speaks for itself.

PART THREE: Appendices

Appendix I: Cooking Tips and Recipes

I continue to discover and develop new recipes, that make low carb cooking a joy. So many are delicious, satisfying, and healthy. There are so many recipes out there that it would be redundant for me to present a list of my own, as they are often presented in a cookbook. That is, as a finished dish, picture perfect with its garnishes, as it would appear at a gourmet restaurant. I don't know about you, but the food I make at home is not as pretty, visually.

I want foods that remind me of the dishes I've always enjoyed, adapted to be compatible with the HFLC diet. So I've taken a slightly different approach at this stage of the book, which is where recipes normally go. Instead of finished recipes, I've compiled a series of tips. Instead of telling my readers how to make a keto-friendly pizza, I present ideas to make a keto-friendly pizza crust. You can make your own pizza the way you like it. The idea is to provide enough alternatives that you will be able to take your traditional favorites, and adapt them so they are keto-friendly, yet still give you that sense of comfort. And at the end, I've compiled some sites you can visit, and browse for recipes.

Bread Alternatives

I used to love a good bread, whether baguette, or rye bread in various styles. And I missed it more than any other food when I gave up flour. And I almost published this book with the lament that you simply can't make anything close to real bread without flour. I had tried most of the types of recipes out there, and found those based on whipped egg whites are dry, and taste like a plastic sponge. Recipes with a lot of almond flour, and varying amounts of coconut flour, come across more as cake than bread. It may be worthwhile for some purposes, but it's not bread.

I came close by starting with fat head pizza dough (covered later), cutting back on the mozzarella cheese, adding some psyllium husk power, and baking powder. It tastes interesting, and is a little

178

reminiscent of bread. The psyllium even gives it a slight yeasty flavor, while retaining moisture inside the loaf. But it never fooled me. It did not even rise properly. Finally, my wife discovered a recipe on dietdoctor.com, and made dinner rolls that I could not tell apart from the real thing, with the caveat that I hadn't had the real thing in over two years. They rose like real bread, and the texture is really convincing.

Details: Mix 1 1/4 cups of almond flour, 5 tablespoons psyllium husk powder, 1 teaspoon salt, 2 teaspoons of baking powder. Gradually add 1 cup of boiling water to the mixture, beating with a mixer as you add the water. Then add 3 eggs, again beating the dough as you mix. Finally, add 2 teaspoons of apple cider vinegar, and mix well. Form the bread or buns as desired, with well-oiled hands, and bake at 350° F for approximately 30 minutes on parchment paper, depending on the size of the loaf or buns.

I've even used this bread recipe to pre-bake a pizza crust, and it makes for a nice alternative to the Fat Heat Pizza Crust, described next. Once the dough is ready, simply use an oiled spatula to spread the dough on parchment paper, and pre-bake for about 10 min, at 350° F.

Fat Head Pizza Crust

For the longest time, I had a pizza craving I could not satisfy. A neighbor, and convert to ketogenic dieting, once offered me a piece of eggplant, topped with pizza toppings, and it was quite good. I experimented with it myself, but soon found it was mostly just a good appetizer. You could not make a whole pizza with it, and pick up a piece with your fingers, the way we're all used to eating pizza. And that was something I continued to miss. Then, I discovered Fat Head Pizza Crust. Take a poll, and some will say it is better than a flour-based crust. It's called Fat Head Pizza Crust, in honor of the movie Fat Head, and possibly originates from a relative of filmmaker Tom Naughton. I've modified it just a little, and here it is, as I make it:

1 3/4 Cups shredded full-fat Mozzarella.

3/4 Cup of almond meal or almond flour (makes no difference)

1/4 Cup of cream cheese

Prepare a 10 by 15 inch cookie sheet (the size that works best for this batch), put a piece of parchment paper on it, and fold the edges of the paper up.

Mix the ingredients in a microwave-safe bowl, and microwave on high for 1 minute.

Mix again, with a spatula, and microwave for another 30 seconds, or up to a minute, until the cheese is soft enough to blend into the other ingredients.

Once the mixture is uniform, and while still warm, add one egg, and mix again with the spatula, until uniform. Spread onto parchment paper with the spatula. The original has you use a roller through a sheet of wax paper, but I could not get that to work very well. For me, simply spreading it with the spatula was much easier. Stretch it to the corners, while careful to seal any tears that form. Make sure it is on the parchment paper, and not directly on the pan, or it will stick irreversibly.

Bake for 8 minutes at 425, high up in the oven, or until brown on top. Remove from the oven, grab the edges of the parchment paper, and flip the crust upside down. Remove the parchment paper, and bake for an additional 5 minutes, or until brown. Until you get the hang of it, with your oven setup, you'll need to watch carefully, so you don't burn it.

Remove from the oven, and make your pizza just the way you want it. Then, put it back in for another five minutes or so, to melt and brown the cheese.

My favorite is to fry up bacon, and using the fat, fry up sliced mushrooms, green and red peppers, and finely chopped celery. I coat the crust with marinara sauce, add the fried vegetables, and cover with full-fat Mozzarella. On top of that, I add pepperoni and crumbled bacon, and sometimes tomato slices. Remember that the crust is already done, so don't burn it. But, if the edges of the crust burn, relax. Just trim them off later. It's delicious, and often preferred over any other pizza. You can eat it like conventional pizza, you can eat it cold, and it also re-heats well.

Also, try using the bread recipe above as a pizza crust, and compare the two.

Crackers

Simply bake the Fat Head pizza crust, but stop the bake a little early, so the crust is only beginning to brown. Slice up the crust, and fry the pieces in coconut oil.

Zucchini Fritters

Other summer squashes may be substituted, with little difference. A single zucchini has about 6 grams of total carbohydrate. But a single zucchini does not go very far, so eat this sparingly. I make it for my family as an occasional alternative to French fries, which I no longer give them.

Grate 2-3 zucchinis into a bowl, depending on how many people there are to feed, and add a teaspoon of salt. Mix well, and let it sit at least 15 minutes. The salt sucks the moisture out of the grated zucchini. Once floating in a deep puddle of moisture, rinse with water to remove excess salt. Don't worry, the water will not quickly re-hydrate the zucchini cells.

Next, squeeze the water out of the rinsed zucchini. Options include layering between paper towels, or putting it into a sieve, and applying gentle pressure.

Add a couple of teaspoons of coconut flour. Just enough that the texture becomes grainy, as the coconut flour absorbs all free water.

Add shredded cheddar cheese in an equal volume to the zucchini, and mix thoroughly. In a microwave-safe bowl, briefly heat the mixture until the cheese is melting, and mix thoroughly. Once sticky, form pancake sized patties by hand, as thin as you can, and fry them in coconut oil. Remove once they start to brown.

Pasta Alternatives

The first pasta alternative is zoodles. Using a spiralizer, such as the Veggetti Spiral Vegetable Slicer that has supposedly been advertised on TV (I don't watch broadcast TV, so I am unaware), spiralize zucchini into strands of approximately ten inches in length. Heat two tablespoons of olive oil to medium-high, add garlic, and fry the zoodles for 2-3 minutes, until soft and beginning to brown. Simple, yet tasty way to accompany foods with sauces, but the noodles themselves should not be the centerpiece. Best to keep it to the equivalent of about one zucchini per person.

The second pasta alternative is spaghetti squash. Slice in half, place face down on a cookie sheet with olive oil, and bake at 350 (Fahrenheit) until fork-tender. Let cool enough to handle safely, and scoop out the strands of spaghetti squash, which will have a noodle-like character.

I prefer the zoodles over spaghetti squash. Despite being acceptably low-carb, I find spaghetti squash to have an unpleasantly sweet taste (but I must admit, after so long, I find dilute lemon juice has a slightly sweet taste). However, if baked into a casserole with plenty of fat, in the form of cream and cheese, the sweetness tends to get lost in the dish.

The final possibility is to make a fat-head pizza crust, and after baking, slice it into strips. This takes a little more work, but the resulting product is more like real noodles, again without the carb.

Alternative to Breading

I grew up regularly eating breaded pork loin schnitzels, and the family has learned to love them. But bread crumbs are out. I learned early that the dense coating they form packs a lot of carb in a small space. Then, when I went carb-free, I desperately wanted a good alternative. But at first, nothing seemed to work. Coconut flour tastes chalky, and almond flour is kind of bland. Frying schnitzels naked is not satisfying. But with a little experimenting, my wife came through with a recipe that tastes a little different, but is so delightful, nobody asks for it with bread crumbs, anymore.

1/2 Cup blanched almond flour (almond meal doesn't stick as well)

1/2 Cup powdered parmesan cheese

1 teaspoon onion powder

1 teaspoon garlic powder

1 teaspoon guar gum

Pre-mix this mixture. If used often, keep a large stock.

Mix two eggs with 1/4 cup of water in a bowl, whipping it up with a fork. Season your favorite meat with salt and pepper, and dip in the whipped egg mixture. Place the meat on a plate with the bread-free mixture, and coat generously. Pat down the coating to firm it up, and let sit for at least 10 minutes. This makes the coating stick to the meat. Fry in coconut oil until golden brown.

The family is happy with it exactly like that, but I am careful to limit my protein, and boost my fat. So I take the finished schnitzel, and melt my favorite cheese on top, with a minute or so in the microwave.

Fixing Lean Meat

Too often, it seems like the centerpiece for a meal is a lean meat. And my definition of lean has changed of late, so even if it is a well marbled steak, I still consider it lean. Too much meat will result in excess protein being converted to glucose, and activate the insulin response, so I limited how much I will eat. The trick is to always leave the table satisfied, having consumed sufficient fat.

The simplest way to fix lean meat is to make a fatty sauce to go with it. My favorite is to fry up baby portabella mushrooms, sliced into big chunks, and once toasted on at least one surface, add a healthy helping of sour cream, some shredded parmesan cheese, or other, milder cheese, some garlic powder, and if it turns out too thick, some heavy whipping cream. The big chunks of mushrooms have a hearty, meaty feel to them, and the sauce is very satisfying. One way to add complexity to its flavor is to add some Thai fish sauce as the mushrooms are being fried. At first, the smell is strong, and even unpleasant, but those flavors soon evaporate, and what remains is subtle, yet very flavorful.

Another favorite is blue cheese sauce. Crumble blue cheese, and add it to a pan with olive or avocado oil, until dissolved. Add sour cream and heavy whipping cream, until it reaches a desired consistency. The tangy flavor of blue cheese goes extremely well with many recipes.

These options, plus a vegetable such as steamed broccoli, can transform a small piece of lean meat into a keto friendly meal that leaves me very satisfied.

Mashed Potato Alternative

If prepared with enough fat, mashed cauliflower can make you forget about mashed potatoes forever. The key is getting in enough fat, and many who have tried simply mashing cauliflower abandoned low-carb eating before they ever gave it a chance. Steamed, mashed cauliflower by itself is horrible. But with a little tinkering, it can be made exceptionally good.

The first step is to steam one medium to large cauliflower, until well over-cooked. It needs to be soft to the touch of a fork. Then, mash it with a fork, or masher, whichever is more convenient. The next issue is that it will be very wet. The easiest way to deal with that is to return it to the hot burner, now off. The excess water will quickly boil off. Once that is done, add 1 cup of sour cream to the mash, about two thirds of a cup of cream cheese, and blend it in using a hand-held blender. A regular blender will also work, but makes cleanup more complicated. This should blend the cauliflower bits to a smooth cream.

Add salt, pepper and garlic powder to taste, and if you want to thicken it a little, some shredded mozzarella. Too much and it becomes stretchy, so stay under 1/2 cup. Mix by hand, until the cheese has melted. Now, transfer to a casserole dish, top with some cheddar cheese and crumbled bacon. Bake in a pre-heated oven at 350° F, until brown on the surface. I'm willing to bet nobody on the standard diet has had cauliflower this good.

Lasagna

There are a million different recipes for lasagna. So pick your favorite, and simply substitute thinly sliced summer squashes for noodles. Unlike other pastas, where the noodle itself is the centerpiece, a lasagna is dominated by the ingredients you choose to add, and the noodles are largely structural. The use of squashes matches the overall flavor of a lasagna perfectly, and indeed some conventional lasagnas include zucchini or other summer squash. You can even include a layer of eggplant, for extra variety in the taste. If you have a favorite recipe you want to adapt, review it first, to ensure that high carb ingredients are not sneaking in. Lastly, when choosing meat, remember to use the cheaper, high-fat ground beef.

Thickening Soup

As soon as I discovered Psyllium husk, I started to try it everywhere that flour might otherwise be used. Soon, I tried to thicken a soup I made from leftover broccoli that was now too soft to eat as a side dish. I blended it, and chopped up some beef tri-tip leftover, added some chopped turnip, a few chopped carrots, and celery. I spiced it with some beef base, and some Thai fish sauce (relax, it mellows nicely as the soup simmers), which adds some complexity to the taste. Anyway, I wanted the final soup to be thicker, so I added a heaping tablespoon of psyllium husk powder to a big pot of soup. That was a big mistake. When I tried to serve it, what started as a very tasty soup became gooey, and highly elastic. Almost rubbery. My kids weren't interested, while my wife laughed that it was like *Ublek*. My analogy was much worse. I waited until she had finished eating, and a while longer for it to settle in her stomach, and only then asked how she enjoyed the *snot soup*. Seriously, it hung off the spoon just like the real thing. It was even green, from the broccoli. I knew at that point that nobody would ever eat it again, so there was no harm in having a laugh at my expense.

The upshot was, she saved the pot, and put it in the fridge. Maybe there was something we could do to fix it, was the thought. The next day, I had the thought that the psyllium probably had nothing else to stick to, so it formed these mucoidal globs. If I gave it something else, maybe it would break up the globs. So I diluted the soup (wife found it a little salty), and added oat fiber. I let it boil, and found it much improved. More oat fiber, boil a while longer, and the rubbery feel was almost completely gone. I had saved the soup. Lesson learned: Psyllium can thicken, but it needs to stick to something else, or it will not be pretty. Oat fiber works, at about two parts oat fiber to one part psyllium.

Later, we learned of a simpler way to thicken soups and sauces. Simply dissolve equal portions of Guar gum and Xanthan gum in olive oil, in a saucepan, and add to whatever you want to thicken. This is used very widely in the food industry, as it turns out. And throwing in a couple of eggs, then whipping them up as the soup boils, is always a good way to add a little extra body.

Smoked Salmon

It is more accurate to say *cured salmon*, or gravlax, which I used to love on a bagel with cream cheese, and a little sliced onion and tomato. Then one day, I decided to simply try it without the bagel, to see how it works. So I sliced some tomatoes, put a slab of cream cheese on each tomato slice, a little red onion, and a piece of gravlax. It was delicious, and is now a standard appetizer. I sometimes put a leaf of fresh basil on top, for good measure. The tomato slice serves as the platform, and it looks as good as it tastes.

A word about how salmon is cured. It is covered with a paper towel, and then covered with salt and sucrose, or sugar. Yes, that bad thing. But it does not taste sweet, unless you mistakenly buy a variant that ruins it by bathing it in honey, without the paper towel as barrier. What the sugar and salt do is suck the water out of the salmon. It's called osmosis, and water always goes to whichever side holds it better. And salt and sugar hold water extremely well, as well as being bacteriostatic. So relax, the sugar does not enter the salmon in appreciable amounts.

Stuffed Jalapeno Peppers

Simply slice the peppers in half lengthwise, and clean out the insides. Slice as big a chunk of cream cheese as will fit inside. Wrap it with a half-length slice of bacon, tucking the loose ends under the pepper. Bake for 30 minutes at 350 F, cool, and serve. This finger food is the first to go at parties, and the jalapeno loses most of its punch, so it only tingles slightly.

Atlantic Salmon

I had nearly given up on skinless Atlantic Salmon fillets, with past experience informing me that they would come out dry, and not very tasty. A shame, because Salmon is a good, fatty fish, rich in omega-3 fats. But one day I was faced with a bag of ageing spinach, and wondered what I might do with it. That's when I found a fantastic recipe on tasteaholics.com, a web site with an extensive list of keto recipes, and a worthy bookmark on any keto dieter's computer.

After thawing and seasoning the salmon fillets, one simply fries up mushrooms, sliced tomatoes, and minced garlic on olive oil. Once the mushrooms are ready, and the tomatoes properly denatured, add in a whole bag of spinach, a bit at a time, until it denatures, and then add more. This vegetable mixture will require added salt, and pepper does not hurt, either. Once done, transfer to a bowl, and drizzle a little balsamic vinegar on the mix. Cover that while you do the salmon.

The web site has you fry the salmon on olive oil, but I wanted a crisper texture on the surface, so I went with a lot of butter, mixed with a little olive oil. Turn the heat up to close to high, and fry the salmon for 3-5 minutes, until crisp on the bottom, and the sides are starting to turn color. Flip, and fry for another 2 or so minutes, until crisp. You have to be quick with this part, to avoid burning the salmon, but that quickness creates a crisp exterior and a soft, buttery interior.

Plate the vegetables in the center of a plate, and place the salmon fillet in the center. It looks beautiful, and you quickly realize this is how salmon was meant to taste.

Mexican Dishes

Tortillas have too much carb, and low carb tortillas (6-8 grams each) taste like the sawdust they contain (actually oat fiber, but it's the same thing). My answer: Don't use them. Once you've finished cooking dinner, and made traditional tortillas for those family members who continue to eat some carb (reduced, but not ketogenic levels), take some shredded cheddar cheese, and sprinkle it on a frying pan. As it is melting, assemble your tortilla on the surface, and fold or roll the resulting food as you like. A simpler version involves melting a layer of cheese directly on the plate, in the microwave, and assembling the other ingredients on top of that.

Desserts

There's no point speaking of dessert unless it is sweet. So dessert alternatives come down to sugar alternatives. Some sugar alternatives are listed below, and we have produced some excellent desserts using them, almond and coconut flours, a lot of cream cheese, heavy whipping cream, coconut oil, and cocoa powder. Cheesecake, almond cakes, brownies, and even home made ice cream can be delicious, occasional treats for the family, without putting the slightest dent in nutritional ketosis.

Keto-Friendly Chocolate

Cocoa has a lot of compounds that promote healing of the circulatory system, so it's something to want. But the sugar in chocolate makes it a no-go. My solution: Make my own. The first thing you need is some raw cocoa butter. I find it necessary to shop on-line to get that. Next, put about 1 1/2 cups of cocoa butter (visual guess, it's hard to measure accurately) in a glass measuring cup, together with a half cup or so of coconut oil. Heat the mix in the microwave, and stir until it all melts. Top up to two cups with coconut oil, and the residual heat should melt the whole thing. Put the melted oil in a mixing bowl. Add 1 1/2 cups of cocoa powder, sifted through a sieve to break up any clumps. Add a half-cup of powdered milk (I grind it in an extra coffee grinder, to smooth the texture), Whisk if up, add a dash of cinnamon (try to use authentic Ceylon cinnamon), a half-teaspoon of vanilla extract, and a few drops of almond extract. Pour it into a cooking sheet with a liner of parchment paper. Ideally, place the tray into a larger one, with ice-water in the larger one. Let it set, then place the tray in the refrigerator for 4 hours, to harden properly. It will have a lower melting point than conventional chocolate, because of the coconut oil, so store it in the fridge. If you take it out of the fridge right before eating it, the consistency is perfect. Experiment with proportions of cocoa butter and coconut oil. The more coconut oil, the lower will be the melting point.

Sugar Alternatives

The mere taste of sweetness can play tricks on the insulin response, so it is important, when beginning the journey to health, to lose the taste for sweet food entirely. That said, on some occasions, dessert is unavoidable. I haven't tried to explain to my children that they can't have birthday cake, because daddy is treating his diabetes. But neither will I allow dessert-levels of sucrose to enter into our diets. I also do not approve of artificial sweeteners such aspartame, acesulfame, cyclamate, or sucralose for my family. So here are some all-natural alternatives.

Stevia. The leaf of the stevia plant tastes very sweet, if you chew on it. The extract has an extremely high specific sweetness, and is sold as a liquid extract, or a powder stabilized with erythritol. A little bit of stevia tastes very much like sugar. A lot of stevia tastes a little bitter, or some say like licorice. For most people, excessive amounts of stevia are unpleasant. Being so sweet, stevia does not add bulk to a dessert, so something is missing. For these reasons, it is best to use in combination with another sweetener.

Erythritol is called a sugar-alcohol, although it has no properties in common with ethanol, so do not be frightened by the word alcohol. Its is simply a class of organic compound. It comes as a granular solid, like sucrose, although it is slightly less sweet. It adds bulk to food. It is absorbed by the body, but is inert when inside the body, and is excreted in the urine a short time later. At high amounts, erythritol is said to produce a cooling sensation on the tongue, although I only experience this if I put some granules directly on my tongue. In moderate amounts, it is used quite successfully in combination with stevia extract, to produce some fine desserts.

Xylitol. Those with dogs should avoid xylitol at all costs. The dog's metabolism cannot tell it apart from sugar, so it produces excess insulin, which can kill the dog by inducing hypoglycemia. Its properties are similar to erythritol, but it tends to produce intestinal bloating, and for me, diarrhea. I do not use xylitol.

Inulin. This is not a typo; it does not say insulin. Inulin is called an oligo-fructan, a small chain of fructose units that is not digested, and is therefore inert in the body. It is not very sweet, but it adds bulk to food, is sticky if trying to create a nut bar, for instance, and caramelizes well. It can be a useful addition to mixtures of erythritol and stevia. But do not use inulin for baking. It can break down at high temperatures, which could release single units of fructose, and that would be very bad.

Monk Fruit Sweetener. The sweet compounds in monk fruit are called *mogrosides*. They are as sweet as stevia, but without that bitter aftertaste. The sweetener is known to lower blood glucose, as it stimulates insulin secretion, without adding any carb load. Due to the high specific sweetness, it is usually formulated with erythritol or inulin. Sounds good? Possibly, but I have reservations about regularly activating insulin secretion. On the other hand, it is the best tasting sugar alternative, when formulated with erythritol. Used occasionally, it is probably fine.

Appendix II: Diabetes Drugs and Supplements

It would be disingenuous of me to pretend I first reviewed the merits of each existing diabetes drug, and only then decided how to combat diabetes. My decision was much more primal. The moment I perceived I was being poisoned by something I was eating, I stopped eating it first, and asked questions later. That said, it is worth reviewing the various classes of drugs used to treat diabetes, their mechanisms of action, and their limitations. In many cases, a working knowledge of the details of glucose transport (covered in Chapter 2) will be valuable to understanding the mechanism by which each drug is intended to work.

The drugs are divided between those that have the objective of stuffing ever more glucose into cells, to get it out of the blood stream, versus those that act by other means (the minority). Once glucose is inside cells, medical thinking declares victory, and is not interested in other problems the strategy may create. In particular, heart disease risk does not improve when a diabetic uses drugs to stuff glucose into cells, and brings blood glucose under control. That says the real risk is what happens to glucose after it is stuffed into cells.

A second point to consider is that when adverse outcomes are reported in connection with a drug, what follows is a give and take between regulators and the pharmaceutical entity. The potential benefits of the drug are weighed against the risks of leaving the disease untreated, and compromises are reached. And when a plausible case can be made that a particular side effect is attributable to the underlying disease, the drug is usually given the benefit of the doubt. I know, we've all seen those commercials listing so many side effects, pronounced so quickly that you think they're irrelevant, or that every sneeze is reported. To an extent, that's true, as the pharmaceutical entity does not want to be accused, in a lawsuit, of hiding possible side effects. But when the disease itself can hide side effects, that becomes a different matter. Please note that this is not an indictment, *per se*. Weighing benefits against risks seems to be a reasonable approach. But it is unlikely we will ever know the full spectrum of side effects of a drug, when the disease itself is associated with those same symptoms.

1. Drugs That Stuff Glucose Into Cells

Metformin

Marketed under the trade name of *Glucophage*, metformin has long been the first choice to treat type II diabetes. Its mechanism of action is by the direct stimulation of AMP kinase, the primary sensor and effector of the cell starvation response. This results in enhanced glucose uptake by the muscles and liver, and decreased glucose production by the liver. Common known side effects are digestive distress, including intestinal cramps, diarrhea, and flatulence.

But metformin should not be mistaken for an insulin-booster. In Chapter 2, I reviewed the two principal signals that cause glucose uptake in liver and muscle. Insulin is one, and the cell starvation response is the other. Both stimulate glucose uptake, but beyond that, they have very different functions. After all, feast and famine are direct opposites.

Metformin causes glucose to accumulate in liver and muscle cells, who think they need to make energy, and quickly. Those cells are instructed by the AMP kinase signal not to make glycogen, or fats. Faced with an ever increasing glucose concentration, the cells may in the extreme ferment that glucose to lactic acid. This can result in a recognized condition called lactic acidosis. From the cells' perspective, that's preferable to allowing glucose to accumulate inside the cell, causing oxidative damage, and cell death. The oxidative stress produced by excess glucose can cause GGT to be released by the liver, which is the single best predictor of an early death.

Further, the underlying condition of insulin resistance will be exacerbated by the increased intracellular glucose level, and the activation of the glycosylation response, which is programmed to limit the levels of intracellular glucose. So the back door around insulin resistance offered by metformin intensifies insulin resistance.

Insulin stimulates the production of fat, where AMP kinase stimulates its breakdown. In a health body, buildup and breakdown each occasionally come into play, but then recede, and allow the other to restore balance. But chronic treatment with metformin tips the balance in favor of breakdown, and over many years, will change the makeup of the body. Muscle wasting, for instance, which may be dismissed as due to age or diabetes, is predicted to worsen.

So is it better to allow blood glucose levels to remain high, rather than take metformin and lower them by stuffing more glucose into cells? It's best to do neither, and instead eliminate the root of the problem.

In addition to metformin, berberine is a natural compound, available as a supplement, that appears to act in the same way as metformin, by activating AMP kinase. It is less well characterized, and therefore carries unknown risks.

Sulfonylureas and Meglitinides

Sulfonylureas and Meglitinides are drugs that stimulate increased insulin production by the pancreatic beta cells. Sulfonylureas have been in use since the 1950s. Produce more insulin, and the existing level of insulin resistance can be overcome, at least for a time. These drugs are capable of stimulating too much insulin production, and causing hypoglycemia, so patients must closely monitor their glucose levels.

There are additional concerns. First, higher insulin levels, in the face of a constant excess of carbs, only leads to increased insulin resistance. Eventually, too much glucose is taken up by cells, which respond by converting some to glucosamine. That activates another pathway to insulin resistance, in turn leading many doctors to raise the dosage of these drugs. This strategy further amplifies the positive feedback loop of increasing insulin resistance, and insulin production. Positive feedback always ends in a decisive manner, since there are inherent limits to how much two processes can amplify one another. A happy example of positive feedback is the contractions that lead to childbirth. An unhappy example is the death of the pancreatic beta cells, from amyloid buildup. That person becomes insulin dependent for the rest of his life.

Untreated type II diabetics already have abnormally high circulating insulin levels, and these drugs will only cause further increases. High insulin levels cause the kidneys to retain fluid, and vascular smooth muscle cells over-proliferate, squeezing harder on the arteries they surround. Both of these factors exacerbate the problems of high blood pressure that always accompany type II diabetes. Then there's the elevated risk of cancer when insulin levels are very high for a long time.

Thiazolidinediones

Doctors make it easy for themselves, and call these compounds *glitazones*. These drugs are activators of a transcriptional regulator known as PPAR-gamma. It is a protein that stimulates a subset of genes. And the genes activated by the glitazones encode proteins that are involved in glucose and lipid metabolism, as well as inflammation. Administration of the drug seems to stimulate all three. Inflammation doesn't get as much press as it deserves, but it is very relevant. It is an inflammatory response that stimulates the production of the protein phosphatase PTP-1B, which turns off the insulin receptor. It is inflammation in endothelial cells that results in the type of thrombosis that precipitates heart attacks and strokes. Inflammation appears to be required for cancer cells to invade surrounding tissue.

The glitazones are able to lower blood glucose without increasing pancreatic insulin secretion, because they force cells to compensate for insulin resistance. But there are concerns. Insulin resistance is a physiological response, and one of its causes is too much glucose uptake, as cells cannot cope with chronically high glucose levels. And the glitazones override the cell's defensive response against excess glucose uptake. If the liver is forced to eat all that glucose, it will labor overtime to turn the excess into fat, thus raising triglycerides and VLDL, and possibly leading to fatty liver disease. Some of the early glitazones were removed from the market because they were toxic to the liver, and the newer ones are being watched closely for any similar effects. It is fair to ask whether any drug that overcomes insulin resistance, in the face of excessive glucose consumption, might pose the same risks. Further, there appears to be an elevated risk of heart failure associated with these drugs. Two factors may come into play. One, increased liver stress caused by increased glucose load results in elevated GGT, and general oxidative stress. Two, gene expression patterns will change in cells all over the body, and cardiac cells might not like those changes.

194

DPP-4 Inhibitors and GLP-1 Analogs

Glucagon-like peptide-1 (GLP-1) stimulates the release of insulin from pancreatic beta cells, but only lives for several minutes in circulation, before it is degraded by DPP-4. So if DPP-4 can be inhibited, GLP-1 can live for a longer time in the blood. That leads to more insulin production, for a longer period of time, and thus better blood glucose numbers. DPP-4 inhibitors exist in pill form, so no injections are needed. But what else does DPP-4 break down? At this point, we don't know if there is anything else, or what consequences there could be to elevating that *anything else*. Caution is called for, until clinical experience catalogs all adverse reactions.

An alternative way to increase the GLP-1 signal is to inject patients with an engineered form of GLP-1 that is no longer susceptible to breakdown by DPP-4. Several of these drugs are now in use, and are quite effective at the narrow goal of reducing blood glucose levels. If I have a concern with this approach, it is that the factor that is normally made for a brief period after a meal, and spends only about two minutes in circulation, now circulates for much longer. Possibly as long as a week. Is this not going to have consequences? One consequence that has been openly discussed is pancreatitis, as the beta cells are worked extra hard. However, as pancreatitis is often a complication of diabetes, the argument that it is caused by the drug is immediately met with, "But those people would get it anyway." The truth is more complicated, and a few simple experiments are not going to give us the full story.

As with the sulfonylurea drugs, use of these agents to stimulate pancreatic beta cells to make more insulin further amplifies the positive feedback loop of increasing insulin production, and insulin resistance. And it also causes more amylin production, which will eventually form amyloid plaques, and accelerate the death of beta cells.

And while these agents will increase blood insulin levels, they do nothing to reverse insulin resistance, or the biochemical problems associated with too much glucose inside cells.

PTP-1B Inhibitor

In the course of my research, I came across a compound called CCF06240, an inhibitor of the protein phosphatase PTP-1B. It has long been known that PTP-1B is a principal inactivator of the insulin receptor, so in theory, if you can inhibit PTP-1B, you can boost the insulin signal. But it is only a numbered compound, meaning it has not been developed as a drug. Compounds generated in early stages of research may be used in laboratory tests on isolated cells, but have a long way to go before they can be drugs on people, and the odds are stacked against it ever getting that far. The same function is available from a component of cinnamon, that has been used a long time. Either way, PTP-1B plays other roles in cells, not least of which is limiting the activity of growth factor signals, which carries an obvious cancer risk. I would be nervous about chronically turning off PTP-1B.

2. Drugs That Remove Glucose From the Body

Drugs that either cause glucose excretion in the urine, or prevent its uptake in the gut, have the potential of improving on the outcomes of those drugs that simply shove it into cells. While an improvement over the drugs that force-feed cells with glucose, these ones accomplish the same thing as is achieved by avoiding glucose consumption, except with the possibility of side-effects. Would you rather eat it and then treat it, or not eat it to begin with?

SGLT2 Inhibitors

Most nutrients in the blood enter the small filters in the kidneys, known as nephrons, but are then reabsorbed into the blood, while urea is excreted. Glucose is one such nutrient, and the protein responsible for re-absorption is called sodium-glucose transporter 2 (SGLT2). GLUT2 does the same thing, but is more widespread in the body. Drug inhibitors of SGLT2 block the re-absorption of glucose in the kidney, where it instead passes through the urinary tract. In addition to lowering blood glucose, these inhibitors are known to reduce blood pressure. They act as diuretics, which can, over the long term, cause the depletion of certain key minerals. Also, urine has plenty of fertilizer, as far as microbes are concerned. Add some glucose, and you have a recipe for bacteria and fungi to overgrow the urinary tract. Over the long term, this poses risks in excess of a few urinary tract infections. Still, this approach has the potential to reduce blood glucose, in the face of excessive glucose consumption, without shifting the problem into individual cells, or amplifying the positive feedback loop.

Alpha-glucosidase inhibitors

To the extent that the diabetic is eating starches (in bread, rice, potatoes) rather than sugars, then those starches have to get broken down to single units of glucose, which can be absorbed in the digestive tract. If this is slowed, or blocked, then the rise in blood glucose levels will be blunted. This class of drugs is the functional equivalent of eating fewer carbs, even while eating more carbs. As such, it does not worsen the underlying condition of diabetic insulin resistance. Of course, leaving that rich a source of energy in the digestive tract means that other micro-organisms are going to use it.

Officially recognized side effects include gas, and intestinal distress. I haven't seen any reports describing the long-term effects on the makeup of intestinal microflora. That is, there are always going to be germs in the intestines. But there are healthy germs, and there are not so healthy germs. If there are even subtle changes in intestinal microflora, over a long period of time, it can raise the risks of various diseases, from inflammatory conditions to cancer. It is not clear whether they would be reported as side-effects of the drug, or because the patient is diabetic, as things that "would happen anyway."

Bile Acid Sequestrants

Bile acid sequestrants were conceived as a way to lower cholesterol, which is an essential component of bile. It is secreted from the gall bladder, but normally reabsorbed from the intestines. By mechanisms that are not well understood, meaning we have no clue why it works, the sequestration of bile acids also lowers blood glucose levels. I'll offer a possible explanation: With bile acids not being reabsorbed, neither will dietary fats. Their presence in the intestines will mimic what happens on a high fat low carb diet, where insulin levels are low, and bile secretion is reduced: Appetite is suppressed, and the person simply eats fewer carbs.

Summary: The majority of diabetes drugs work by force-feeding cells more glucose, thus removing it from the blood. Victory is declared, and we do not ask what happens to that glucose afterwards. But the toxicity of glucose is not unique in the blood. It is even more toxic in the reducing environment of the cell, where oxidative damage can be severe. This is the leading possibility to explain why aggressive reductions in blood glucose do not improve cardiovascular disease, and may actually make things worse.

Drugs that boost the secretion of insulin risk all of the above, plus they accelerate the rate of pancreatic burnout, at which point, the patient will require insulin injections.

Another class of diabetes drugs interfere with the breakdown of starches in the gut, or prevent glucose reabsorption in the kidney. In both cases, carb-rich waste product passes through the system. The best that can be said for these drugs is that they mimic the act of avoiding dietary carbohydrates entirely.

Natural Products That Lower Blood Glucose

In addition to the products of chemistry and/or biotechnology, there are natural products that can reduce blood glucose levels. Some are known to be effective at reducing blood glucose, but the risk profiles are not well characterized. Natural products cannot ordinarily be patented, and when a product is not owned by someone who can make a lot of money off it, nobody is willing to invest in characterizing it, and learning its plusses and minuses. Much of the research done on natural products today comes from China, which has a long history of using natural compounds in traditional medicine. Some supplements have true pharmaceutical properties, and are inexpensive alternatives to patented medicines. But simply because something comes from nature does not automatically make it healthy, or effective, just as being artificial does not mean it is inherently bad or good. So caution is in order.

Cinnamon

Cinnamon is able to inhibit PTP-1B, the main down-regulator of the insulin receptor, and one probable agent of insulin resistance. Some would go so far as to eat several grams of cinnamon with each meal. But be careful. Nearly all the cinnamon on the market is the

Cassia variety, and is distinct from the more expensive true cinnamon, that only comes from Ceylon (Sri Lanka). Both have the anti-PTP-1B property, but *Cassia* also contains significant amounts of coumarin, which when consumed over the long term, is toxic to the liver. I've seen reports that the European Union has ordered bakers to phase out *Cassia*, which is expected to raise the price of cinnamon in Europe.

However, coumarin is fat soluble, whereas the compounds that inhibit PTP-1B are water soluble. It is possible to buy water extracts of cinnamon, that have the active compounds, but lack the coumarin. Keep in mind that cinnamon is likely to work by a pharmaceutical mechanism. It forcibly suppresses insulin resistance, and coaxes the cell to consume even more glucose, against its consent.

Cinnamon will reduce the blood glucose of many who are insulin resistant, and probably will not improve the diabetic risk of heart disease, since the glucose is still there, only it has been stuffed into cells.

Corisolic Acid

Extracted from banaba leaf, corisolic acid has long been used to lower glucose, and a large body of research supports its use for that narrow objective. There are suggestions that it works by activating PPAR-gamma, which would make it a cheap alternative to the glitazones, but in theory, it will also carry similar risks. I've also seen suggestions that it is a PTP-1B inhibitor. In either case, it is another pharmaceutical-like natural product, that shoves ever more glucose into cells.

Alpha Lipoic Acid

This is a true dietary supplement, in that it does not work by pharmaceutical means. It is naturally present in mitochondria, but seems to be reduced in diabetics. As a supplement, it is known for anti-inflammatory properties, improving insulin sensitivity, and stimulating fat burning. It is approved in Germany for the treatment of diabetic neuropathy, where it requires a prescription. Anywhere else, it is not officially approved, but is available without a prescription. Is there any logic here?

Chromium Picolinate

There are reports that it can lower blood glucose, but if taken to excess, chromium is toxic. It is present in leafy vegetables at safe concentrations, so it might be best to simply regularly eat lettuce, spinach, or kale.

Gymnema Sylvestre, Korean Ginseng, Astragalus Root

Used in Ayurvedic medicine for countless years, gymnema consists of leaves from a common vine in India. Plenty of evidence suggests that it can lower blood glucose levels, but some reports suggest it can elevate blood pressure. Likewise Korean Ginseng. Astragalus is supposed to lower blood pressure, but sporadic reports suggest it can raise blood pressure. Accordingly, it is best to proceed with an abundance of caution.

Diabetics need to be wary of conflicting reports, where a drug or supplement is said to help blood pressure, where other reports suggest it worsens symptoms. Diabetics are metabolically different than other people, and may react differently as a consequence. Those who stop consuming glucose and carbohydrates in any meaningful quantity are also anomalous, because a lot of metabolic changes occur as the body adapts to burning fats instead of glucose.

Lastly, the mechanisms of action of these supplements are not characterized. Supplement makers don't generate enough revenue to justify funding expensive science, so we may never have that information. I'm not against these supplements being available, but we should be cautious when we lack information.

Vitamin D

Vitamin D is the sunshine vitamin, because it is converted to its active form (vitamin D3) in the skin, by the action of sunshine (although it is also available in supplement pills). Vitamin D was discovered as the factor that could prevent rickets, the malformation of growing bones, if 400 units or more were consumed daily. As a result, 400 units was enshrined as the necessary daily dose. Case closed. How about the other functions of vitamin D? *We already know it prevents rickets, so don't complicate our lives*, might be the medical community's response.

Units are defined arbitrarily, so a large or small number means nothing without context. And twenty minutes of full sun, such as at the beach in a swim suit, will produce (estimates vary) between 20,000 and 50,000 units of vitamin D3. Why would the body produce so much, if it only needed 400 units, and only in youth, while bones were growing? The answer is, because it boosts the immune system, helps fight infections, cancer, and other diseases.

There are also numerous reports implicating vitamin D deficiency in worsening the severity of heart disease, and yes, diabetes. I have benefited from much less severe respiratory infections while taking vitamin D for many years, but I still came down with diabetes. So vitamin D is obviously not sufficient to protect against diabetes.

Magnesium

After experiencing the keto flu, where minerals arc a little out of whack, I added a magnesium supplement to my daily routine, knowing that most people are deficient in the mineral, and that deficiency is associated with high blood pressure, and various forms of cardiovascular problems. Magnesium is an essential co-factor for a lot of essential processes. It's not good to bc lacking it. And I should add that most magnesium supplements are useless at actually increasing the blood levels of magnesium. Magnesium oxide is the cheapest form of magnesium, and is sold both as a chalky laxative, for which it works, and a supplement to raise blood magnesium levels, for which it does not work. An effective magnesium supplement has to be *chelated* magnesium. That means the magnesium ion is surrounded by other chemical entities, to make it soluble and easy to absorb. Apparently, a lot of people have discovered this, and shifted their buying preferences to chelated magnesium. The problem is, it is much more expensive for the manufacturer. Supplement manufacturers seem to have clued in, and invented a new term, *buffered* chelated magnesium. The buffer is the chalky magnesium oxide, but they assure that *some* of the magnesium is chelated. How much, they usually won't say. On-line reviews of those products are riddled with negative reviews, written by people who've discovered the deception, and eager to give them a piece of their mind.

Winnowing Down

In the early stages of my recovery from diabetes, I experimented with metformin for about a month, and possibly saw a modest improvement at first, but eventually decided it was no longer doing anything for me. I was improving with our without it, so I discontinued its use. I continue to take alpha lipoic acid, because of its role in treating neuropathy. I experimented with many of the supplements listed above, and despite my best intentions, could not bring myself to conduct proper, controlled experiments when my health was on the line. I dropped some when I was having blood pressure problems in the early days. I'm not about to go back and see which ones might cause the same problems.

Supplements such as alpha lipoic acid, vitamins B, C, and D, and magnesium are things the body needs, and deficiency can cause disease. Then there are extracts that do not directly impact blood glucose control, and are not strictly necessary, but stimulate healing from the damage caused by diabetes. Pine bark extract is often cited as a stimulator of microvasculature re-growth, and grape seed extract seems to contain the same compounds at a lower cost. Turmeric seems popular, and in a test tube, the compound curcumin has some attractive looking properties. Criticisms are that it's poorly absorbed, and quickly excreted, but it does bind up iron in the gut, helping to protect against iron overload, a common problem for men, and post-menopausal women.

It's a worthy goal to want to eliminate the need for diabetes drugs. And with the exception of injected insulin, for those who lack their own, all can be eliminated by healthy eating (fat, not carb). But I can't advise anyone on *how* to get there. I never took any drug that stimulates insulin secretion, or potentiates its action. With those drugs, hypoglycemia is always a danger, so care is needed to balance carb reduction and diabetes drug reduction, and eventually, elimination. Between your doctor's guidance, and your own experience, you will need to find a safe way to eliminate them, without risking hypoglycemia.

Appendix III: Further Resources

On Cholesterol, Carbs, Obesity:

Books:

Good Calories, Bad Calories, by Gary Taubes (the definitive work)

The Cholesterol Myths, by Uffe Ravnskov, MD PhD

The Great Cholesterol Con, by Dr. Malcolm Kendrick

Fat Chance, by Dr. Robert Lustig

Cholesterol Clarity, by Jimmy Moore and Eric Westman, MD

Taubes also wrote a simpler version of the story that I have not read, titled: *Why We Get Fat, and What to Do About It*

Short Videos:

Cholesterol and Heart Disease, by Malcolm Kendrick (Youtube code i8SSCNaaDcE)

Sugar: The Bitter Truth, by Robert Lustig (Youtube code dBnniua6-oM)

Why We Get Fat, by Gary Taubes (Youtube code lDneyrETR2o)

Enjoy Eating Saturated Fats: They're Good for You by Donald W. Miller (Youtube code vRe9z32NZHY)

Movies:

Sugar Coated You'll never reach for the white, deadly stuff again

Fat Head Laugh and be educated by one irreverent movie

On Ketogenic Diets, and Recipes:

Keto Clarity, by Jimmy Moore and Eric Westman, MD. Perfect introductory work.

The Ketogenic Cookbook, by Jimmy Moore and Maria Emmerich. Keep it near your kitchen.

The Keto Diet, by Leanne Vogel. Another cookbook. I haven't read it, but it has excellent reviews.

Online recipes:

These sites will show recipes, free for your taking, but most also sell cookbooks. If you like their recipes, please consider supporting them by buying a cookbook. And I expect there will be many others. As you explore online, you will find no end of quality resources to support the keto lifestyle.

https://www.tasteaholics.com/

https://www.ruled.me/keto-recipes/

https://ketodietapp.com/Blog

https://www.dietdoctor.com/

https://elanaspantry.com/diets/keto/

http://www.wickedstuffed.com/

Appendix IV: Data Presentation

For those in officially metric countries, this may come as a surprise, but mg/dl is actually a metric unit. There is nothing non-metric about it. It is not, however, any longer the officially approved unit as mandated by the metric cops. My glucose meter is American, so it gives me a reading in mg/dl. The round number of 100 mg/dl separates good from suspect blood glucose readings. Remind me again why Celsius is such a good measure of temperature? Oh, never mind. Here is how to convert units: To convert mg/dl to mM (same as mmol/L), divide by 18. To go back, multiply by 18. The following table does it for you.

mM	mg/dl	mM	mg/dl	mM	mg/dl
0.28	5	6.7	120	16	288
0.55	10	7	126	16.6	300
1	18	7.2	130	17	306
1.5	27	7.5	135	18	325
2	36	7.8	140	19	342
2.2	40	8	145	20	360
2.5	45	8.3	150	20.8	375
2.8	50	8.9	160	22.2	400
3	54	9	162	23	414
3.3	60	9.4	170	24	432
3.9	70	10	180	25	450
4	72	10.5	190	26.4	475
4.4	80	11	196	27.7	500
4.7	85	11.1	200	30	540
5	90	12	216	33.3	600
5.5	100	12.5	225	38.8	700
6	106	13.9	250	40	720
6.1	110	14.4	260	44.4	800
6.4	115	15	270	50	900

To interpret an HbA1C reading, here is a table that attempts to match predicted average glucose levels, relative to A1C measurements:

HbA1C level	Estimated average blood glucose level
5 percent	97 mg/dL (5.4 mmol/L)
6 percent	126 mg/dL (7 mmol/L)
7 percent	154 mg/dL (8.5 mmol/L)
8 percent	183 mg/dL (10.2 mmol/L)
9 percent	212 mg/dL (11.8 mmol/L)
10 percent	240 mg/dL (13.3 mmol/L)
11 percent	269 mg/dL (14.9 mmol/L)
12 percent	298 mg/dL (16.5 mmol/L)
13 percent	326 mg/dL (18.1 mmol/L)
14 percent	355 mg/dL (19.7 mmol/L)

Glossary

Acetyl-CoA: Metabolic intermediate. It delivers fuel from the breakdown of sugars, fats, and proteins to the citric acid cycle, used to generate cellular energy.

Adipocytes: Fat cells, below the skin.

AMP: Adenosine Monophosphate. The product when cellular ATP stores are depleted.

AMP Kinase: Sensor of AMP accumulation, meaning the cell is in danger of starving. It triggers alarms, and stimulates responses to quickly restore cellular energy levels.

Amylin: Hormone produced in a rigid proportion of 1:100 with insulin. The higher insulin goes, amylin goes up with it. Too much amylin can damage pancreatic beta cells.

Anaerobic: Without the use of air. It refers to glucose fermentation without oxygen.

ATP: Adenosine Triphosphate. The principal energy store of the cell, built up by burning or fermenting fuel, and used by all metabolic processes.

BHB: Beta hydroxybutyrate. The principal blood ketone. It serves as an energy source for certain parts of the brain during periods of fasting, or carb avoidance. Low levels are healthy, but it is best known for ketoacidosis, where its levels are out of control.

Carbohydrates: All forms of sugar, whether in single units, or large chains. Strictly speaking, includes alcohol.

Cellulose: Chain made of glucose units that is very stable, and not easily digested. Only herbivores can use it for energy.

Chylomicrons: Vesicles that transport fats from the gut to fat cells. Also known as ULDL.

Corticotropin: Hormone made by the pituitary gland, that triggers the adrenal cortex to release cortisol, the stress hormone.

Cortisol: The stress hormone, but also plays a role in waking up, for example. Has many functions in the body.

CRH: Corticotropin releasing hormone. Made by the hypothalamus in response to stress. Triggers the pituitary to release corticotropin. Drugs exist that block the CRH receptor.

Cytokines: Hormones used by the immune system to coordinate an immune response.

Endocrine: Hormones injected into the blood, to regulate parts of the body. Insulin is an endocrine factor, and endocrinologists see a lot of diabetes patients.

Endothelium: Like skin, except on the inside of the body, rather than the outside. Endothelium is the lining on the inside of blood vessels, for example.

Fibrinogen: One of the principal factors involved in the formation of blood clots. High fibrinogen is the single biggest risk factor for heart disease.

Fructose: The sweet sugar. It is also very reactive, and toxic. The liver is the only organ that can process it, and quickly overloads. It then has to convert it to fat.

GGT: Gamma glutamyl transferase. A marker of liver stress, and cause of oxidative stress in the blood. Used by insurance companies as the best single marker of death risk.

Glucagon: Hormone produced by the alpha cells of the pancreas. It tells the liver to make new glucose. When alpha cells become insulin resistant, glucagon is elevated, and glucose is too.

Gluconeogenesis: Making new glucose. The liver uses amino acids from protein breakdown, and turns them into glucose. It is why high protein is essentially high carb.

glucosamine.

Glucose: The least reactive simple sugar, and usable by all cells in the body.

GLUT: Glucose transporter. Specialized proteins that shuttle glucose into cells. Only GLUT4 is controlled by insulin at all, and insulin is only one of several signals that can activate GLUT4.

Glycerol: A metabolite of glucose, used to make fats into triglycerides. Fats are free to move in or out of the cell. Triglycerides are not.

Glycation: The reaction of glucose with another molecule, often a protein. It happens by itself, without any specialized enzymes. It releases reactive oxygen, and damages the thing it reacts with. It is why glucose is toxic.

Glycosylation: A small amount of glucose in a cell is converted to glucosamine, which is attached to proteins by specialized enzymes. It acts as a glucose sensor, and inhibits insulin action in multiple ways, to limit glucose toxicity.

Glycogen: Chain of glucose units stored in animal cells. It is easily broken down, to make glucose available.

HbA1C: The percentage (or molar concentration) of hemoglobin that has been glycated by glucose. It serves as a marker of average blood glucose over the past few months, and a proxy for glucose damage.

HFCS: High-fructose corn syrup. A mixture of glucose and fructose, used widely as a sweetener.

HFLC: High-fat low carb. Do not confuse with HFCS.

HPA Axis: The regulatory network of hypothalamus-pituitary-adrenal cortex. It is the mediator of the stress response.

Hyperglycemia: High blood glucose.

Hypertrophy: Overgrowth. Something that has grown beyond healthy measures.

IGF-I: Insulin-like growth factor-I. The mediator of the effects of growth hormone, but the receptor can also be activated by elevated insulin. May also play a role in the progression of cancer.

Incretins: Pancreatic hormones that stimulate the release of insulin.

Insulin: The signal to make and store fat. Taking up glucose and storing it only when it is in low supply.

Ketone: A molecule produced by metabolizing fat, for use by certain parts of the brain when glucose is not readily available.

Ketoacidosis: A dangerous condition experience by those with no insulin of their own. Glucose and the ketone BHB are both very high.

Ketogenic: A diet that deprives the body of glucose, so it produces ketones. The amounts are well-controlled, so long as even a little insulin is available.

Ketosis: A state where a part of the body's energy needs are met by ketones. Fasting, or low-carb dieting produce ketosis.

LDL, pattern A, pattern B: Two very different blood lipid particles, but both fractionate in the zone known as LDL. Pattern A are large particles, considered harmless. Pattern B are small, hard, sticky, and prone to oxidation. They are considered dangerous.

Leptin: A hormone made by fat cells, telling the brain they are satisfied, and don't need to be fed. Insulin resistance causes leptin resistance, and obesity follows.

Lipase: An enzyme that breaks up triglycerides into fats and glycerol. Hungry cells make a lot of lipase. Full cells do not.

Metabolic Syndrome: The combination of diabetes, obesity, high blood pressure, and bad blood lipid profiles that always seems to occur together.

High insulin is the common factor.

Microvasculature: The network of small blood vessels, where the exchange between blood and tissues happens. It is easily damaged by high blood glucose.

Mitochondria: The cell's energy factories. They burn acetyl-CoA, and make ATP. If something goes bad in the cell, the mitochondria trigger a self-destruct sequence.

Saturated fat: Fat holding as many hydrogen atoms as it can. It cannot be further hydrogenated.

Secretion: Something squirted into blood, or digestion, by a specialized gland.

Starch: A chain of glucose molecules, made by plants, that can be fully digested into glucose molecules in the human gut.

Sucrose: A binary sugar, of one unit of fructose and one unit of glucose, joined together. In the gut, it is converted to the equivalent of HFCS in seconds.

Trans fat: A type of unsaturated fat produced by artificial hydrogenation, that is not recognized by the cell's mitochondria, and gums them up.

Triglyceride: Three fat molecules joined to one molecule of glycerol. Cannot cross cell membranes, so it can be stored stably in fat cells.

Unsaturated fat: Fat molecules that can be hydrogenated, because they have room for extra hydrogens. Monounsaturated fats have only one place where extra hydrogens can be added, whereas polyunsaturated fats have multiple places. More prone to oxidation than saturated fat.